Phone 22

FREEPORT, N. S. _July 21_ 19 54

Freeport N.S.

IN ACCOUNT WITH

J. CAMERON MacDONALD, M. D., C. M.

	TO PROFESSIONAL SERVICES AND MEDICINE		
ay 15	Delivery 1 Baby	25	00
un 1	Additional House Calls — measles.	3	00
uly 10	Sammy — Broken Wrist	10	00
	X-Ray	5	00
	Total	43	00

THE ISLAND DOCTOR

Memories, myths and musings of a country doctor

J. Cameron MacDonald MD

Published by Princess O'Toole Press
840 Argyle Road, Windsor, Ontario, Canada N8Y 3J9
www.princessotoole.com

Library and Archives Canada Cataloguing in Publication

MacDonald, J. Cameron (John Cameron),
The island doctor : memories, myths and musings of a
country doctor / J. Cameron MacDonald.

ISBN 978-1-897509-04-3

1. MacDonald, J. Cameron (John Cameron)
2. Medicine, Rural–Nova Scotia–Digby (County)–Anecdotes.
3. Physicians–Nova Scotia–Digby (County)–Biography.
4. Long Island (Digby, N.S.)–Biography.
5. Brier Island (N.S.)–Biography. I. Title.

R464.M234A3 2009   610.92   C2009-902292-3

Design by Hydesmith Communications
Printed in Canada on 100% post-consumer recyled paper by Friesens

Dedication

This small volume is dedicated to 1,200 of the world's most wonderful people, who live on the islands of Digby County where I spent five of the happiest years of my life. I thank you all for giving me the honour and privilege of being your country doctor for the most interesting and rewarding experience every young medical graduate could hope for.

It is also dedicated to country physicians everywhere, in the hope of encouraging and perhaps stimulating an interest among graduating physicians to consider going into medical practice in a rural community... to experience the enjoyment, the fun, satisfaction and pleasure of having your patients be your neighbours, confidants and best friends.

It is really a wonderful life.

J. Cameron MacDonald MD

THE ISLAND DOCTOR

Memories, myths and musings of a country doctor
J. Cameron MacDonald MD

Acknowledgements

It has taken 57 years, the longest gestation period in history, to produce this small volume. Successful accomplishment of this great feat is due to the contributions of a number of people. Among them, my younger son, Michael, who, on hearing these stories over and over, insisted that every person has a book in him or her, but also complained that all the interesting memories of our family happened before he was born.

"So why were they not written down?" he asked, giving motivation to the project.

My daughter, Betts, provided inspiration, ideas and misplaced memories. Betts was my last obstetrical (emergency) home delivery before we left the Digby Islands. I always maintained that she was my original do-it-yourself project and that she and I were the only sensible and logical members of this family.

Betts's husband, airline pilot Bill McClinton, rescued me every time I screwed-up a computer program.

My elder son, Cam, a master storyteller and business advisor, was involved in most of the yarns in this book and was most helpful in recalling lost details.

Katie, my wife of 59 years, to paraphrase Winston Churchill, had the courage to marry me and the stamina to stay with me – and loved me more than I ever deserved to be loved.

Katie, the reason for any and every success I have ever had, "lived and loved life on the islands, contributed, and even manufactured memories.... and then demonstrated remarkable tolerance and fortitude over the many years of re-telling and embellishing of these stories ("fables" according to Terry MacLeod).

My editor, Rick Johnson of Final Copy Editorial Services (www.finalcopy.ca) in Winnipeg, Manitoba, applied his expertise in organizing, editing and providing constructive suggestions for production, printing and marketing of this great work of mixed fact and fiction. Rick's tolerance of my many changes, re-writes and other foibles is much appreciated.

And finally, my wonderful, persuasive and persistent daughter,

Ellen, also in Winnipeg, and her husband, radio broadcaster Terry MacLeod, gave great encouragement and support... Terry insisting I should pay more attention to fact than fiction... but where's the fun in that? Ellen, through her company, The Perfect Publicist (www.theperfectpublicist.com) put this whole project together, cajoling, bullying and threatening me until I cooperated in doing my part to get it finalized. *(This is an unsolicited testimonial from a loving father.)*

Foreword

From my very first encounter with Cam MacDonald almost thirty years ago, I quickly learned four essential things about him: he loved being a doctor, he adored Katie, he was a gifted storyteller, and he was obsessed with two remote islands in the Bay of Fundy. The first three things were evident to me – I could see them with my own eyes every time I had the pleasure of his company. But those islands? Where were they, really? What was it about them that cast such a spell on him? Cam told me his stories about them so often that I could recite them too: Arthur and the furniture; Clyde Stark and the snow storm; Katie and Princess O'Toole; Odessa and the baby. But I had never heard of Brier and Long Island before I met Cam.

(That's not technically true. Growing up in PEI and playing as a kid with the grandchildren of Angus Walters of Bluenose fame, I had heard of that other great Nova Scotia sailor, Joshua Slocum, who was the first person to sail around the world alone. He too was a legendary figure and, no co-incidence, had been reared at Westport on Brier Island.)

The magical way that Cam talked about life in Westport and Freeport and Central Grove made me wonder if the islands were just his version of that mythical musical village of Brigadoon. Had they and their larger-than-life inhabitants appeared out of the mist to Katie and Cam once long ago and then vanished forever?

In the summer of 2008, Cam insisted that my son Finn and I travel with him and Katie to visit this flesh-and-blood "Brigadoon". And it was all true... well, mostly true. We trekked around the fog-wrapped coastline of this miniature world at the end of Digby Neck and saw Arthur's house, called Clyde's son, and tracked down that baby born at Odessa's. We even saw Joshua Slocum's shack.

Perhaps it was the fog, or maybe it was the rum, but in those few days the magic of the place began to settle on me too. Boats and herons and whales and storytellers emerged from the fog and, without a moment's notice, vanished. Had I seen them or just imagined them? The intersection of fact and fiction was somewhere in the fog where Brier Island's Northern Light was blinking. There was something about this place and these people that required yarns and tall tales to describe them. And, when I quizzed Cam as to whether his stories were all true, he replied in classic Brier Island style: "Why let the facts get in the way of a good story?"

Enjoy your time in the fog on Cam's "Brigadoon". I know I did.

Terry MacLeod
Winnipeg, November, 2008

Preface

As a kid growing up in the steel company town of Sydney, Nova Scotia, on Cape Breton Island, I had heard and read about the wonderful lives of country doctors, in particular, how that short, fat wrinkled and rumpled little physician had delivered, cared for and saved the Dionne quintuplets. And how horse and buggy doctors struggled through snow storms to save lives with mustard plasters and the dispensing of things like Burdock Blood Bitters to make people strong and healthy, and gave sulphur and molasses to kids every spring to clear their systems of all the debris that collected during the winter months. They doled out Dodd's Kidney pills because, "They do the work of calomel, but have no calomel or mercury in them." I marveled at Carter's Little Liver pills, which also did wonderful things.

My life, on the other hand, seemed relatively dull. Sure, my father was a lawyer, city solicitor and Member of Parliament, but nothing exciting seemed to be happening. My brother and I went to Sacred Heart School and, with 15 or 20 other kids, delivered newspapers for the Sydney Post Record at noon. We had been taught by the nuns to whisper "Blessed be the name of Jesus" any time we heard the Lord's name taken in vain but there was so much profanity yelled by the kids clamoring for their bundle of papers for delivery that my brother and I, continuously muttering, "Blessed be the name of Jesus," acquired the reputation of being the most profane of all the kids.

We lived in a big house and mother had a series of maids, one of whom was from Newfoundland. She was with us several years and after she left, mother, clearing up her room, found a letter the maid had written home. It said, in part, "They lights candles here and goes to Mass, but I just laughs it off."

Father's very good friend, Reverend Alexander A. Murray, was a Presbyterian Minister. He was a very nice man and we all liked him. Reverend Murray recorded his sermons to be broadcast over CJCB Radio every Sunday morning. Our family would go to Mass then come home to listen to the Presbyterian radio sermon.

In the early days of radio, primitive recording and replaying were often not reliable. On one Sunday morning, Reverend Murray thundered out: "Are you a true blue Presbyterian? A true blue Presbyterian is one who has placed his worldly goods at the feet of the Lord Gee...Gee...Gee... Gee bxbxbxbxxkee... KEEKHRIST." My brother and I thought this hilarious but father felt we all should be more sympathetic and understanding, especially toward a man trying to spread the word of God.

In retrospect, I realize there were religious differences at the time but they never bothered the multinational kids of mixed backgrounds and colours in our neighbourhood. They all seemed like normal kids just having fun playing ball in the backyard next to the Chinese restaurant (one of my father's best clients).

During one such game my brother hit a home run right through the second storey window of a house owned and occupied by a bald-headed, one-armed bootlegger. The kid who pitched the ball was the son of that bootlegger, also one of my father's clients. The man was annoyed and very articulate as he bellowed profane and politically incorrect comments about race, colour, religion and illegitimacy. The kids quickly retreated to what we called Pelican Beach.

The Pelican was an old, rusting iron British navy ship, sunken at the wharf and heeled over at 45 degrees. It had a huge mast with a rope dangling from the crow's nest. It was great fun to grab the rope on the high side of the ship, swing out and drop into the polluted water of Sydney Harbour, then swim back to the ship and climb up the ragged, rusty iron deck to get another turn. Kids got scratched and bruised but, miraculously, never seriously hurt or infected – another wonder of self preservation of kids.

The stories in this book recall the escapades of a young country doctor with the supreme, if unfounded confidence of youth, anxiously going into medical practice in an isolated, rural community. The stories are mostly true, allowing for minor memory lapses, of course, a touch of creativity, and a modicum of embellishment. It must also be acknowledged that truth is to story telling as gin is to chastity.

I hope you enjoy reading them as much as I have enjoyed retelling them.

CHAPTER ONE
Sydney Academy

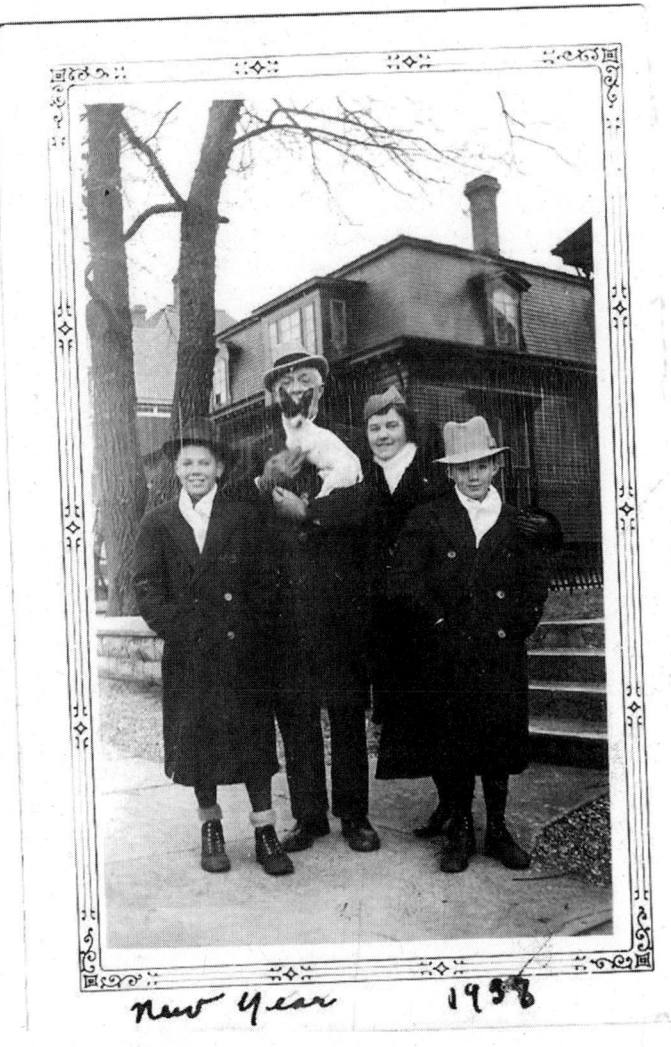

New Year 1938

The high school principal called a failing Grade 12 student into his office. The kid was depressed, sulky; he had low self esteem, perhaps due in part to his severe acne.

"You have been in this school for three years," Mr. Campbell said to the boy, "and you have failed every grade. We thought you had promise and promoted you each year hoping you might improve... you didn't!

"The teachers are disappointed in you," he went on. "Your parents... your father a lawyer, your mother a teacher... are disappointed in you; you're a disappointment to yourself and to your friends. In the history of Sydney Academy there is only one academic record worse than yours... that of your older brother and I expelled him two years ago. Now I am expelling you."

The kid's older brother, taller, athletic and confident, had lots of friends and not a trace of acne. He was better at everything than his kid brother and now even surpassed him on the list of disgraced students of Sydney Academy. Not only that, but their mother also liked the older brother best!

The year was 1942, the third year of the Second World War. The skinny, expelled kid was defeated and lonely in a crowd. He had no direction, no ambition, and though he had a good home with concerned parents, he had no idea what he wanted to do with his life. Others his age and older were in military uniform so he went to the recruiting station of the Cape Breton Highlanders Regiment. There he met a large, muscular, abrupt and arrogant army sergeant with a bulky mustache and hostile attitude. The sergeant looked at the insecure, sunken-chested kid with severe acne and growled: "Go away kid... come back when yer growed up."

The only other "opportunity" available was employment at the steel company division of the Dominion Steel and Coal Company. To that point the kid's memories of his father's often taking the family to the steel plant in their 1925 Oldsmobile Touring Car to eat ice cream and watch the dumping of slag into the tar pond constituted the only knowledge he had of the place. To the kid, those had been exciting excursions; the colours were beautiful and the outings created happy family recollections.

In the 1930s, the environment was not even a consideration

but today that same tar pond is considered the worst industrial contamination site in all of Canada.

Most able-bodied men in Sydney were in uniform. DOSCO needed all the labourers it could get and were even willing to hire a skinny kid. He was assigned to the open-hearth department and told to get a shovel from the tool shed.

Each of the four open-hearth furnaces was 40-50 feet across the front and 15 feet deep. Molten steel was processed in each furnace and when ready, the huge furnace was tilted backwards to spill the white/red hot steel into large iron vats waiting on the railway tracks below, then rotated back to its base. The labour gang then pitched shovelfuls of dolomite, a fine, white gravel, to the back of the furnace where the molten steel had been. This process required the ability to throw one's shovelful, in one bolus, 15 feet to the back of the furnace and smartly get out of the way of the next man, while using your shovel to shield your face from the intense heat.

The next man up would throw his bolus immediately beside the previous one until the entire back wall was covered. Novices like the skinny kid had to learn the technique of keeping the bolus of dolomite together instead of spraying it around the furnace. Any skill is worth learning and eventually the kid mastered this one, joined the union, and became an accepted member of the team. He got to like his fellow workers and, although they were all older and bigger and called him "kid", he was able to carry his share of the workload.

Occasionally, members of the labour gang were picked out to do other tasks. The kid was told one day he was to become be a welder's assistant. The job was on the roof over the open-hearth furnaces. It consisted of spot welding corrugated, galvanized sheets of steel (four- by eight-foot panels) onto steel girders. The kid's job was to help slide the panels into place for welding.

The kid was scared of heights and that high above the ground he was terrified; one leg tightly wrapped around a girder was not much help. The welder was an experienced roofer, a young, tall, lean, fit, nonchalant and happy fellow. He laughed at the scared kid while he slid a panel into place, fitted it, spot welded four corners and reached for another panel. With the grace of a ballet dancer, he then leaped to the next girder. The kid was amazed at the agility and confidence of a man so unafraid and so good at what he did. He became a hero to the kid but the kid, clinging to a lonely girder, remained an almost completely useless helper.

The heat and soot from the open-hearth furnaces made the roof hot and dirty but the work progressed and, nearing completion, the welder reached for the last panel. It was caught on something and, standing on an open girder, he jerked it free but lost his balance in the process. For a long moment the welder, holding onto the loose but slipping steel panel with his right hand, vainly flailed his left in an attempt to regain his balance. The kid let go of his grip on the girder and grabbed the moving panel but was not strong enough to hold it. The welder fell backwards off the roof, followed by the sheet of steel. The horrified kid watched him fall 75 feet to his death on the railway tracks below. Crying, scared, dirty and frightened, he climbed down the ladder from the roof, his hand bleeding from trying to hold the ragged edge of steel panel.

By the time he reached the ground a large crowd had gathered to see the crumpled body of the welder. The steel company ambulance arrived and the company doctor was called. This was the third year of the Second World War and everything was rationed, from sugar and coffee to gasoline. Automobile production was severely restricted and only medical doctors were permitted to buy new cars. The steel company doctor drove up in a brand new Buick sedan, the biggest and most beautiful dark blue car, with polished chrome trim, whitewall tires and leather upholstery. The doctor got out and the crowd separated to let him through. He had on a steel grey suit, white shirt, a blue tie that was the same colour as the car, and even shined shoes. He approached the welder's body and, with a gesture of a clean hand with manicured nails, pronounced to the ambulance attendant: "He's dead, call the morgue wagon."

The kid watched as the doctor walked back to his car and drove away, a professional man, important (The crowd had separated to let him pass). He was undoubtedly rich, driving a brand new car in wartime. The kid's father, also a professional, was a lawyer. His mother, also a professional, was a teacher. Why couldn't he get to be like one of them?

The kid looked at himself... dirty, unkempt, a school dropout, no goals, no future, and certainly no new car! He looked at the welder, a skilled tradesman; the man he had admired and even envied so much up on the roof was now dead at his feet. The comparison was compelling. The kid was 17; a light went on in his brain. Maybe Mr. Campbell was right. Maybe he did have promise, but sure as hell, something had to change.

Humbled and contrite, the kid went back to the school principal and with his guidance and new motivation, enrolled in night school courses in English, history, mathematics, and even auto mechanics, while still working at the open-hearth 48 hours a week for a year and a half, at 45 cents an hour. The principal tutored, guided and encouraged the kid until he was able to earn enough credits to qualify for admission to Saint Francis Xavier University.

At university, life became enjoyable. The kid had friends, he was happy, and his acne even disappeared. University life was wonderful. People, including the kid, had goals and made plans for the future. Teachers, professors and fellow students were interested and interesting. Life was good, better than anything the kid could ever have wished for... but he had a lingering regret that a man had to die to awaken and motivate him.

The kid grew up, became a doctor and practised medicine for more than 50 years. Happily married, he raised a family of four: two boys and two girls, all of whom were sufficiently motivated to become university graduates. He now has seven grandchildren and has owned several new Buicks.

He often reflects on the singular event that changed the course of his life from the sulky, indolent and useless teenaged kid into a productive citizen who, as a physician for 50 years, must have affected the lives of many people. He has often wondered what motivates or stimulates teenagers of the type he had been... and he often speculates on the "what-ifs?"

What if he had not flunked out of high school? What would he have done? What if he had not become a labourer in the open hearth and someone else had gone to help the welder? The other person would have been older, bigger, stronger and probably not afraid of heights. He would have been more help to the welder and the welder might not have been killed... perhaps. In that case, the kid might never have had a sufficiently shocking experience and might never have awakened.

What if the kid had been able to help the welder and the welder had not fallen, and both were able to climb down the ladder without injury? Would the kid have learned anything, or just grown old and still be working as an unskilled labourer in the open hearth.

If the irresponsible kid was the cause of, or even responsible for the death of a co-worker, should he feel guilty even while realizing that same tragedy provided the incentive to change the course of his own life? Now, in the twilight of my life, I know there is no going back, and no resolution to the debate.

CHAPTER TWO

The Digby Islands:
a Voyage of Discovery

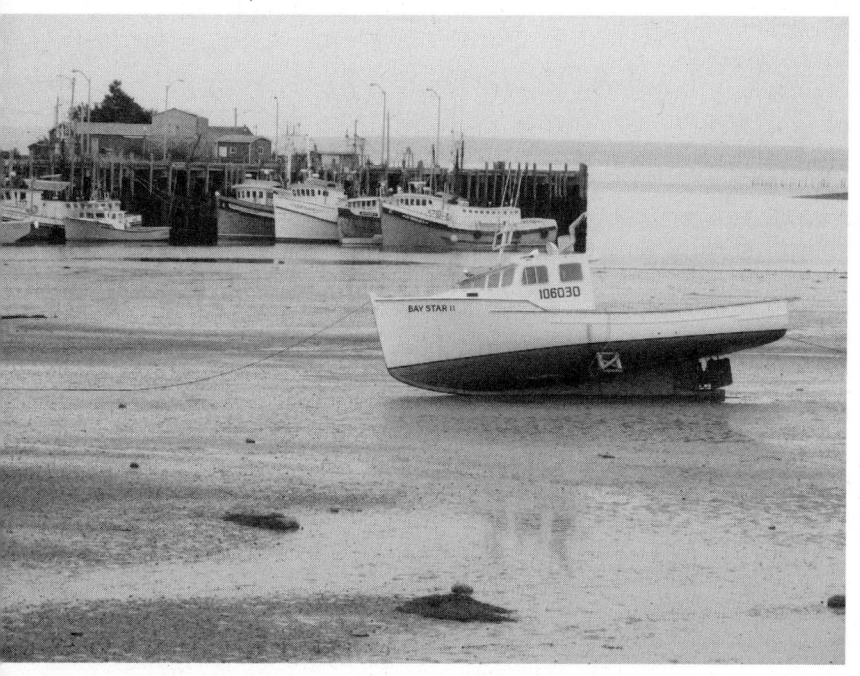

A s an eager young medical student, I dreamed of becoming a doctor, saving lives, being respected and beloved by my fellow man. I had read stories of country doctors in the horse and buggy days and of the wonders of modern medicine in 1951. I just knew I could do it and I thought I could do it best as a country doctor.

During my intern year, I heard about an opening for someone to take over from a doctor who was retiring after 25 years on an island in the Bay of Fundy. I was interested and went to find out more. I learned there were actually two islands and about 1,200 people, all served by that one doctor. The nearest hospital was 40 miles away. With no hospital, no ambulance service or fire department, and only an occasional visit by a policeman, this would be a great place for a newly graduated physician who was absolutely convinced there was nothing he didn't know about medicine, or anything else for that matter. This was obviously the place for an old fashioned country doctor; it would be a challenge and an opportunity for a brilliant young medical graduate to bring modern medicine to the needy. And I just knew I was the one destined to do it.

Three schools, three or four Baptist churches and an IOOF lodge were on the islands. The main and only industry was fishing. Two government-run ferries operated, one ran back and forth to the mainland and the other between the islands. The doctor had a big house with a two-room office. Mostly, he made house calls and had very little office practice. He did 12-15 home deliveries per year.

The Bay of Fundy is a 50-mile-wide diverticulum of the Atlantic Ocean encircled by the coasts of the State of Maine, New Brunswick and Nova Scotia. The tides are the highest in the world, changing every six hours and, depending on the phase of the moon, rise and fall 24-35 feet. When the northeast wind blows in off the Atlantic against the direction of the tidal flow, monstrous waves and other threatening weather conditions develop.

The Digby Islands, Long Island and Brier Island, are at the peripheral end of a 30-mile-long peninsula extending into the Bay of Fundy from the Town of Digby, parallel to the northwestern shore of Nova Scotia.

The Village of Freeport was built around a cove, sheltered from the ravages of the Bay of Fundy. The tide flows into the cove and the 25-30-foot-long fishing boats sail in on the incoming tide, pick up their moorings and waft gently in the protected water. When the tide goes out, the boats rest on the mud flats, providing an opportunity to do repairs, such as painting, caulking and whatever else their hulls needed below the waterline.

Brier Island is a rocky guardian of the most westerly point of Nova Scotia. The Village of Westport is unique. Fishing and tourism and whale watching are the main industries, with two fish-processing plants, beautifully maintained, colourful houses with well-tended gardens and manicured lawns.

The 350 people of Westport are elite, God fearing, interesting people with their own schools, churches, a library and a visiting branch of the Bank of Nova Scotia (every Thursday afternoon).

When I told my Irish Catholic father-in-law I had decided to take his daughter to live and practice medicine on the Digby Islands, his response was both abrupt, definitive, decisive, Irish Catholic, and profane.

"I've been blown ashore and shipwrecked on those Gawddamn islands. There's nothing there but rock, seaweed, dried codfish and Baptists."

Despite his objections, Katie and I were firm in our decision to move to the islands and, much to our delight, my father-in-law came to visit frequently.

Coincidentally, an elderly lady from Tiverton, a village on the island, happened to be a patient in the Saint John General Hospital where I had been an intern. Katie and I went to see her. She was pleased the islands were to have a new doctor and thought it a wonderful place to live and to bring up children because, among other things, "We have no Negroes, no Indians, no Jews and no Roman Catholics."

Katie and I were both born into Irish Roman Catholics families, Katie in Saint John and I in Cape Breton. We had both gone to Catholic schools and always figured this religious separation was just a parental thing and of no concern to us kids so, in our naiveté, and never having understood serious bigotry, we were not offended. We were more amused, surprised, and too green to even recognize the attitude as a potential problem. And it never was.

Fortunately, we were not dissuaded from our decision to settle on the islands. In our five years there, there was never a suggestion of religious conflict. We made many life-long friends and attended church services, funerals and functions in the Baptist Church hall. At the request of the elders of the church, we (two Roman Catholics) even helped the Baptist Church Council decide from a list of applications who should be their new minister.

At one of the funerals, our two small dogs, who happened to be Irish terriers (but with no religious convictions) marched as solemn mourners in the funeral procession from the church to the grave site.

The ceremony included the singing of several hymns by a trio of rather buxom ladies. As they began, first with a pitch pipe, then with "Beyond the Sunset, Oh Grateful Morning...," our two faithful hounds, acknowledging their heritage of arctic wolves howling at the full moon, put their heads back and joined in with loud, protracted, doleful wailing, not far off key from the trio.

Katie and I were embarassed and tried to silence them but they were part of island life and were not about to be disuaded. The mourners, at first shocked, then amused, finally applauded in appreciation of the Catholic canines taking part in the Baptist ceremony.

We were happy to accept invitations to the annual banquet of the IOOF lodge and were always seated at the head table, pleased to contribute to the after-dinner entertainment. Anecdotes from old copies of the Readers' Digest were most helpful on such occasions. It should also be noted that these meetings were always held on a Friday night, with ham and turkey on the menu but, for the Roman Catholic doctor and his wife, who were not permitted to eat meat on a Friday, an elegant lobster platter was always prepared.

Shortly after arriving on the islands, I lost my watch and asked an oldtimer the time, which, I learned later, provided him with an opportunity he relished – to greet in his own peculiar way, another newcomer to the island.

"Sonny," he said, "you ain't been here very long. Nobody needs a watch on the island. You want a page off the calendar?"

With that, as part of his routine, he reached into his pocket and pulled out a calendar page, May, 1951.

"From this you can see when the moon is new and when it's full. When it's new and full, the tide is high at half past nine in the morning and low at half past three in the afternoon. Now," he continued, "from the way the damn government built the ramps for the ferry, you can't get a car on or off this island for two hours on either side of low water, so when the moon is new or full, you're stuck here from half past one till half past five. The tide is three quarters of an hour later every day. The ferry don't run after dark. Your stomach tells you when you're hungry, and what the hell else do you need to know?"

Katie and I loved the island life. We participated in every activity. We even helped build a baseball field and organize a league. We laughed and cried with friends who were also all patients. I even became part of the unofficial police force, frequently called upon to quell a disorderly drunk "with a shot of something." This often required a squad of at least four men to overpower the guy while I loaded a syringe of a compound called "paraldehyde", which, incidentally, is never used anymore but produced eight hours of peaceful sleep, with resulting horrible halitosis. Often, this was enough to make a confirmed boozer take the temperance pledge.

Katie and I made a great team. She helped out at the school, taught sewing lessons to teenaged girls, was my telephone answering service and receptionist, and often came with me to home deliveries, administering the required four drops of chloroform to the mother's mask during labour and looking after the newborn infant. On more than one occasion, when nothing else was available, she even stripped off her petticoat to wrap the babe.

On one occasion, when I was in Tiverton, Katie called Elsie, the telephone operator. Elsie tracked me down with several telephone calls, asking everyone, "Did you see the doctor? Which way was he heading?"

Three men had been cutting logs for firewood when one was hit by a falling tree, breaking his lower leg. His buddies had lifted him onto the back of a pickup truck and took him to our house. He was in severe pain, yelling and crying. Katie asked me what she could do.

"Give him a good drink of rum. I'll be there in 15 minutes," I said.

Katie's mother never tolerated alcohol in her home and Katie had no idea of what "a drink of rum" amounted to.

"Should I give him a teaspoonful?" she asked, to which I barked, "KEE..... RHIST Kate, give him a belter of rum!" and hung up. A "belter" was a Cape Breton term she had not heard. She was confused, standing with a 40-ounce bottle of rum in one hand and a large tumbler in the other. A teaspoonful was obviously ridiculous, so she filled the tumbler and gave it to the guy with the broken leg.

By the time I got there, the man had worked his way to the tailgate of the pickup and was dangling his broken leg over the end and singing bawdy songs. Fortuitously, this was a good position for the fracture. His heavy boot put traction on the leg, separating and aligning the fractured bone fragments, thereby helping to relieve the pain and hold the leg in ideal position.

I got a long extension cord and my portable X-ray machine, X-rayed the fracture right at the tailgate of the pickup, developed the film in my back porch and, with the bones in ideal position, applied a plaster cast... with half the population of Freeport watching and cheering the marvels of modern medicine.

The man happened to be a member of the Baptist Church Council. His wife was shocked and mortified that her saintly, Bible-toting, Sunday-school-teaching husband, a lay reader in the Baptist Church, and within a stone's throw of that church, was singing raunchy, bawdy barroom songs. And what was worse, he knew both the lyrics and the melodies.

She blamed Katie, calling her a shrew, a vixen, a Mary Magdalene who had even seduced her husband with alcohol to bite the apple in the Garden of Eden. But Katie, loved by all the other island folk, had followed doctor's orders, relieved the man's pain, performed a humanitarian service, and was recognized as the hero of the day.

However, the island people made us welcome, even holding a banquet to introduce us to the community. The ladies sewing circle made curtains and drapes; the men helped fix, paint and renovate our house and supplied us with lobster, scallops and fresh fish.

Elsie was an unpaid executive assistant and the ferry boat operators pledged to be available any time, day or night. We were so pleased with the reception we received that I began feeling sorry for my classmates who had gone into urban medical practice.

CHAPTER THREE
Odessa

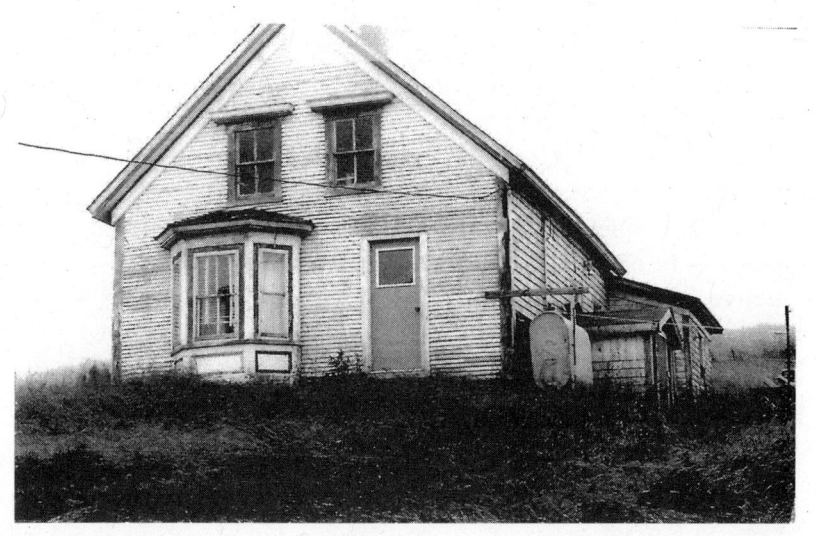

The Village of Freeport on the Digby Islands is a quiet fishing community built around a cove where 20-30-foot fishing boats float in on a high or mid-tide and lie on the sand and mud at low tide. Their owners are then able to repaint and repair them before the next tide.

I had been granted a medical doctor's degree by Dalhousie University just three days before. (Universities *grant* degrees; rarely do they admit one has been earned.)

The nerve centre of the islands was Elsie, the telephone operator. Every telephone was on a party line so Elsie knew everything that went on 24 hours a day. It was 10 o'clock at night when she called to say a woman living at Fish Point was about to "come sick". Not being familiar with the colloquial expression, I needed an interpretation.

It was a "confinement", I was told (another Old World term). "She's having a baby and needs the doctor."

In the modern hospital of that era, I had had the usual intern rotation in obstetrics and though never having attended a home delivery, I knew, with youthful arrogance, everything I could possibly need to know. I had studied the pamphlet put out by the Nova Scotia Department of Health on maternal and child care, including Chapter 3, entitled "Domiciliary Obstetrics".

In hospital, the intern's situation is supervised and simplified. Invariably, there is a veteran case room nurse, who has seen and been a part of every obstetrical complication imaginable and knows what to do about it, what instrument to hand to the arrogant young expert... and what to tell him to do with it.

Home deliveries are different. That young arrogant know-it-all is on his own. Fortunately, I had been befriended by an older doctor who had had experience with domiciliary obstetrics and, in addition to presenting me with his old home "Obs Kit", including almost every instrument I would need, he advised that the fancy new leather medical bag that my mother had presented to me was totally inadequate.

"What you need," he had said, "is a big suitcase, at least 30 by 24 by 6 inches, sturdy and waterproof."

Chapter 3 of the Nova Scotia government pamphlet described

how the instruments should be thoroughly washed and wrapped in cotton cloth, recommending Robin Hood Flour bags, bleached to remove the colour. The package was then to be baked in the oven at 350 degrees Fahrenheit until the cloth appeared scorched – but not burned. That would render the instruments at least surgically acceptable if not sterile.

Added to my suitcase were at least two operating-room gowns, caps, masks and sterile rubber gloves. The anaesthetic of choice for home deliveries in the 1950s was chloroform. Four drops on a mask was sufficient to give very effective relief of pain. My confidence was bolstered by a comment made by one of my mentors that, "In medical practice, as in anything else, you may not be the most qualified person in the world to handle the emergency, but you will be the most qualified one present."

With those words solidly in my memory, I drove to Fish Point. The tide was high and the moon was full, reflecting off the small boats floating in the cove, the fish plant, the ferry wharf, Brier Island, and the lonely fisherman's house where I was about to become one of the major actors in my first independent medical miracle.

I walked up the hill carrying my new fibreboard suitcase and my shiny new medical bag. The weather-beaten, wooden clapboard house was obviously in need of repair. The veranda floor sagged as I walked across it to the door.

The husband, a big powerful man, greeted me. He had a rugged complexion, the result of having spent years of his life on the Bay of Fundy. Odessa was his sister, an equally large woman, who quickly informed me that she had never been involved in the delivery of a baby before and that she was nervous and shivering. Indeed, the little old house seemed to shake with her every tremble.

Two small children were running around and, for reasons I have never understood, the obligatory large container of boiling water was on the wood stove in the kitchen. Just off the kitchen was a room with a double bed... and the woman about to deliver her third child. In a corner of that room was a pot-bellied Quebec heater with a roaring fire and, dangling from the ceiling, a lonely 40-watt light bulb. The rest of the house was in semi darkness.

I set up my instruments on a makeshift table beside the bed, got appropriately dressed in my O.R. gown, cap, mask and gloves, examined my patient and prepared for delivery. I told Odessa to give the patient an enema. This medical terminology required more earthy clarification but having had experience on a labour gang in the Sydney steel plant, I had the necessary vocabulary.

Then, realizing the two urchins were still running around the kitchen dangerously close to the hot stove and the large container of boiling water, I ordered the husband to move the solitary light bulb from my case room to the socket dangling from a wire in the kitchen. To provide light for the delivery I had decided to use the flashlight in my car and went to get it.

After ripping my sterile gown climbing over the rusty barbed wire fence and, as I opened the car door and glove compartment with my sterile, gloved hand and the interior light came on, I realized I might have a problem... little did I know.

On returning to the case room, the enema had been given and the results, in a makeshift bedpan, were placed on top of my sterile instrument tray. When the time came for delivery, I gave the flashlight to a trembling six-foot-one-inch, 250-pound Odessa and told her where to point it. The room continued to shudder with her trembling.

I put four drops of chloroform on the small chrome mask covered with three layers of surgical gauze. It worked well, the labour pain was relieved but the light from my flashlight was waving all over the ceiling. Odessa, holding the flashlight with one hand, was covering her eyes with the other. While still trying to appear composed, in control, and with the air of a commanding officer, I said to her: "God is sending us a little bundle from heaven, so now, for Khrrrrrr...ist sake, shine the light here so He will know where to put it."

Odessa stuttered that she would t-t-t-try. With the next pain, the baby's head was crowning but Odessa, standing immediately behind and over me, had had enough and fainted. In her fall, she inadvertently kicked shut the partially opened kitchen door; the flashlight rolled under the bed; the bottle of chloroform flew out of my hand and smashed against the hot Quebec heater in the corner; Odessa was on top of me and I was on top of the spread-eagled mother with the baby between her thighs, umbilical cord still attached.

I recalled from medical military training that chloroform exposed to open flame makes phosgene gas, the war gas used against Canadian soldiers at Somme in World War I.

I didn't have a "problem", I had a critical situation to deal with! In an almost totally dark room, the only light coming from a sliver of moonlight through a dirty window partially covered by frayed curtains, I had a new baby boy with umbilical cord still attached, and his mother, both in danger of being crushed under my weight, compounded by a 250-pound unconscious body on top of me, while war gas bubbled up in the corner of the room. Immediate action was required and, while not the most qualified person in the world to deal with the situation, I reminded myself that I was the most qualified person present, although I did wonder what my boyhood movie hero, Dr. Kildare, would do.

My surgical instruments were scattered on the floor but the moonlight glinted off something shiny. I reached and found a Kelly clamp and scissors, clamped and cut the cord and shook Odessa off my back. Fortunately, the husband had heard the commotion and came charging through the door. I grabbed the babe, he picked up the mother and between us we managed to drag Odessa by her feet, bloomers and all, out into the kitchen.

I put the babe in the Eaton's mail order bassinette on the oven door, ordered the husband to break the case room window from the outside to release the phosgene, hoping we wouldn't poison the whole village, and went back to look at the babe only to find the plastic liner of the bassinette had caught fire.

I rescued the babe once again and both he and his mother recovered uneventfully and quickly... it took me a little longer.

The village survived and I, with my first home delivery, had brought a new citizen into the world. He was named after me and after such an exciting, grand debut, I knew he was destined for a great and adventurous life.

I made the usual post-natal visits daily for about 10 days, then weekly until I was satisfied all was well with mother and child. The little guy was being well fed, both by breast and bottle, and there were no ill effects from the fire, poison gas or bacterial contamination during delivery.

I did try to impress upon the mother the importance of cleanliness and sterilization of the baby's bottles in the prevention of infantile diarrhea, dehydration and whatever else.

On my monthly visits, the baby was doing very well. One day, when he was about a year and a half old, I was waiting for the Westport ferry and dropped in for a visit. The dad, who had just returned from a shift cutting fish at Connors' Canning Plant, was still dressed in big rubber boots folded below the knee and clothes soaked and smelling of fish guts. The baby was sitting in a carriage holding a bottle and, as the father came in, the baby tossed the bottle out onto the floor. The dad bent to pick it up but inadvertently kicked it into a corner of the room. When he retrieved it, as was the custom, he wiped the nipple off on the seat of his fish-soaked pants and put it back in the baby's mouth.

I followed that baby for five years. He grew, gained weight, thrived and never had an infection or childhood disease. He had been exposed to every local pathogen and obviously developed immunity to them all. It was enough to shake a young doctor's belief in the need for sterility, cleanliness, and the science of bacteriology.

The delivery of this child in 1951 was my introduction to domiciliary obstetrics. It was more interesting, challenging and frightening than any of the multiple other home deliveries I subsequently had on the islands.

I predicted at the time that the new citizen I had just ushered into the world with such excitement and fanfare had to be destined for a great and adventurous life. He was even named after me. When I again met Cameron Albright in 2008, 57 years later, I learned that my prediction had not only come true but that it had also been grossly underestimated. I stand today in reflected glory that I was present at the start of the life of this remarkable man.

At an early age, Cameron became interested in cartooning and, upon completing Grade 12, studied at the Nova Scotia College of

Art and Design in Halifax. He later published a book featuring a copyright cartoon character he created in 1973. That character ran as a cartoon strip from 1982 to 1991. During that period, Cameron also designed and built his first house, with the help and guidance of his older brother, Bill.

As an artist, Cameron prefers to work with water colours but also enjoys oils and charcoal. Boats and sea scenes are his favourite subjects and he takes commission on specific boat paintings. His art work can be found in homes in Canada, United States, Denmark, Sweden, Germany, Holland and different countries in West Africa.

He and his wife, Janis, met in 1971 and life has been an adventure ever since. They moved to Granville Ferry in 1977 where they set up a printing, silk screening and sign painting business. During that time, they also became interested in sailing.

In 1987, they closed the business, took two of their children and left the country until 1992. During those five years they did volunteer work for a non-profit organization called Mercy Ships. They spent a year in Hawaii at the University of the Nations then joined the medical and relief ship Anastasis. They did two trips to Jamaica after hurricane seasons wiped out homes and crops; they helped build a school and homes for people while there.

Cameron entered an officer training program while on the ship and his training and sea time were monitored by ship's officers. While with the organization, they did relief work in the Dominican Republic where they helped build schools for deaf children and, in their spare time, built a house for a shoeshine boy who had won their hearts. They sponsored that boy in a private school so he could become educated.

The ship crossed the Atlantic and then sailed out of Europe and Africa. They were in Berlin when the wall fell, in Estonia when the Russian coup took place, and spent time in Togo, Ghana, Guinea and Ivory Coast. In Ghana, Cameron was invited by a local man to travel inland up the Volga River to visit villages. That was a highlight for him because the people told him he was the first white person to visit and stay overnight. The ship would stop at the Canary Islands to give the crew a break before returning to Europe. The Albrights had a motorcycle and, while with the ship, also did bike trips across France and inland Africa.

They returned to Canada in 1992 because their daughter, Jael, was looking to go to university. Upon their return, Cameron went to the Nautical University in Port Hawksbury where he studied and got his third mate's unlimited tonnage, unlimited, ocean-going ticket. He also studied on his own and was tested for his Captain's ticket for a 350-ton vessel, limited to South America.

After completing these challenges, Cameron and Janis were able to buy Dunromin Campground in Nova Scotia. *(Checkout their website at www.dunromincampsite.com.)* They live in the province from May until October, then cruise the Bahamas on their sailboat, Te Amor, throughout the winter.

They have three children: Jantina, who has two sons, Skyler and Jake, and who resides in Florida and operates her own company; daughter Jael, who has one son, Zachery, and works for IBM, lives in Iowa and is expecting a wee one in spring, 2009; son Joshua works as their manager at the campground and will eventually buy them out and take over when they retire.

At present, they are building their retirement home in Granville Ferry across the road from the home where they raised their family. Once again, Cameron has designed this house to take in the view of the historic town of Annapolis Royal. They have named the house "Waters Edge"; every room except the two bathrooms has a view of the water.

Cameron is a gentle, spiritual soul who loves adventures and meeting new people, especially people from other cultures. Once you have met him you will never forget him. His smile has opened many doors far and wide.

CHAPTER FOUR

Arthur,
the Legend and His Furniture

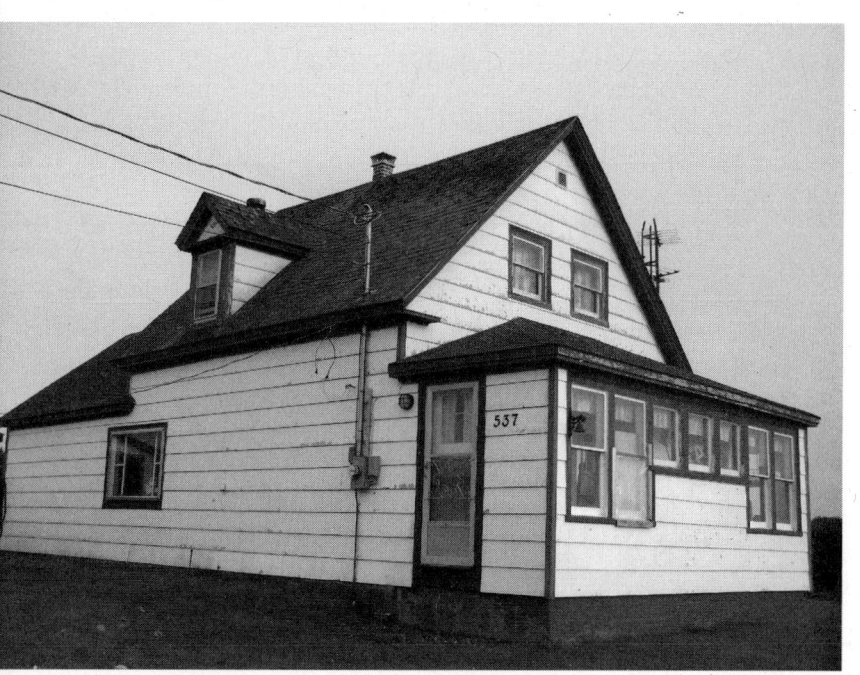

Arthur was a tall, good looking man in his late 40s, dignified, well-spoken though shy, polite and confident. He was a strikingly handsome man with distinctive features, black hair greying at the temples and an air reminiscent of Gary Cooper. His swarthy complexion was typical of a life spent on the Bay of Fundy.

Arthur was embarrassed that he had been ordered by his wife to come to see me. He was cleanly and simply dressed and was tired, pale and "just not feelin' good." The thought of going to a doctor with such a frivolous complaint was not for a macho guy.

I had seen Arthur professionally on only one previous occasion. He had had an abscessed right mandibular molar. The tooth was beyond salvation and had to be extracted. There was no dentist on the island and he was in pain... extraction became my responsibility.

The old doctor I had replaced on the island had instructed me in what to do in this, as well as many other situations. He had also left with me an old pair of universal dental forceps. This instrument resembles a hefty pair of pliers with angled and tapered jaws, ideally suited for the task at hand.

In addition, I was given a mouth gag, a heavy wire device to be placed between the jaws. It had a lever on one side to force and keep the jaws open. Then with my trusty four drops of chloroform, I had approximately 20 seconds of anaesthesia, sufficient time to pry open Arthur's jaws and latch on to the offending tooth.

Now, it should be noted, a tooth is never "pulled", it must be loosened by gentle rocking, which is what I was doing when my 20 seconds of anaesthesia were used up. While I held firmly onto the tooth with dental forceps, Arthur, regaining consciousness, grabbed my wrist with his powerful right hand and, in one forceful move, extracted his own tooth.

The reason for Arthur's "not feelin' good" became apparent very quickly. He was lean, well muscled, but on physical examination I found a tremendously enlarged spleen. A blood count acquired in my very primitive office laboratory showed a massive increase in the number of his white blood cells. The most likely diagnosis was chronic myelogenous leukemia, which demanded immediate medical care.

I called the cancer clinic in Halifax and they agreed to see him the next day. Arthur made the seven-hour, 150-mile trip by bus. The clinic confirmed the diagnosis of chronic myelogenous leukemia and started him on whatever chemotherapy agents were available in 1952. At that time, in the natural history of the disease, life expectancy was estimated to be four to five years. Arthur was treated in hospital in Halifax and sent home on medication, returning to the clinic at regular times, monthly at first, then every two to three months, and eventually at six-month intervals.

Arthur was an ideal patient; he complied with instructions and continued his life as a fisherman. Eventually, his disease caught up to him and after four and a half years, as the cancer clinic specialists had predicted, his defences began to crumble. The cancer clinic had done everything it could and advised him that he should get his affairs in order, and that he had, at most, three to four months left to live.

Arthur, having philosophically accepted his fate during the seven-hour bus trip, felt at peace with the World. He arrived in the Town of Digby and, while waiting for the connecting bus to the islands, saw a large sign in the window of the Digby Home Furnishing store. It read:

Six rooms of furniture $4,000
No money down
No payments for six months
Life insured/no medical exam required
Not even a questionnaire

Four thousand dollars! As a fisherman of very modest means, that was more money than Arthur had ever dreamed of having. As he looked at the sign, he thought how nice it would be to have all that stuff.

He wandered into Wong's Restaurant, had a meal of wonton soup and Digby scallops, apple pie and even a beer. Arthur had been told not to drink alcohol with his medication but with only three months left, what did he have to lose. He came out of the restaurant and sat in the park. It was a beautiful fall day. The leaves were changing colours and the sun was shining brightly on the Bay of Fundy; it was good to be alive.

He reflected on his life and remembered, among other things, the teacher he had had in Grade 8 some 30 years previous. That teacher, a young man he knew as Mr. Olmstead, was just out of "normal school" (Now it's called teachers' college). He was enthusiastic, interesting, and made a lasting impression on students. Arthur remembered him as the best teacher he had ever had.

Mr. Olmstead, Arthur recalled, made history come alive. Among other things, he talked about famous world leaders and how they often had to make important decisions. He gave the examples of Julius Caesar crossing the Rubicon, Lindbergh Crossing the Atlantic, and Washington crossing the Delaware. They had all made decisions that involved risk before realizing their ultimate success.

Arthur, looking at the sign in the furniture store, pondered the biggest decision he would ever have to make. Yes, world leaders agonized over big decisions but he was no world leader, yet he had a big decision to make nonetheless. The doctor had told him he had three months to live, there would be no payments for six months, and all that new furniture would be his. But suppose the doctor was wrong and he lasted more than six months? Well... he could make one or two monthly payments if necessary.

With another beer, it seemed easier to come to a decision. With courage and bravado, Arthur went in, bought six rooms of furniture for his small house for $4,000 with no money down, no payments for six months, life insured, and no medical exam... not even a questionnaire. He then got on the bus to the island, pleased, elated even, happy and comfortable with the thought that he, like other great men of history, had been decisive. He had made an important decision and he was proud of it.

Ten days later, a big truck loaded with Arthur's furniture arrived at East Ferry. It had to wait for several crossings because the ferry was only big enough for four cars and the truck was as large as any four cars.

At 10 a.m., the truck arrived on the island with all the new furniture. By 10:15, the whole village had turned out to cheer. Elsie's information network had sprung into action. By now, everyone knew what Arthur had done. As the island's nerve centre, Elsie knew every bit of gossip, where everybody was and what anyone said about anything. Long before CNN, Elsie was the original EIN – the Elsie Information Network.

As the truck rumbled along the gravel road to Freeport, a motorcade developed and people came out of their houses to wave and cheer. Arthur's house, a wooden clapboard one-storey with five rooms and a loft, was around the cove at Freeport. Arthur had just bought six rooms of furniture and squeezing it in would be a problem. By custom, the entrance to any house on the island was through the kitchen. They all had front doors as well, but since front doors were never used, no one ever built steps up to them. As Arthur's new furniture arrived, the men of the village thought his house deserved to have new steps up to the front door. They found lumber, hardware, and even concrete blocks for a foundation for the new steps. Arthur's house soon became the only one on the island so equipped.

The excitement was palpable and increasing. People from all three villages came by car, on foot, by horseback, wagon, bicycle, bus and boat. One couple arrived in an ox-driven cart. A crew arrived from Halifax's CJCH Radio and Television to do a remote broadcast. This was before the term photojournalism had been coined. They portrayed Arthur and big business as a modern version of David and Goliath.

The Halifax Chronicle Herald ran a front-page headline: "Arthur wins". Victor Cardoza, the colourful and occasionally overly dramatic editor and roving reporter from our local weekly tabloid, The Digby Courier, went even further, likening Arthur to Greek mythology and the legend of Horatio on the bridge, quoting: "How can a man die better than facing fearful odds, for the glory of his fathers and the temple of his gods."

The Acadian Press in Metegan reported the story in French. The Cape Breton Highlands News Bulletin told local and very envious Scots all about Arthur... in Gaelic! The whole world knew about Arthur in at least three official languages.

Under Arthur's direction, the men of the village carried out the old furniture: the old sagging beds and battered bedroom furniture, the beaten up old sofa from the kitchen, even some Eaton's catalogue chairs from the parlor with the plastic still on them. Everything had to go.

This was exciting; six rooms of furniture were to go into a five-room house. The men laid a new linoleum floor in the kitchen. The women of the village pitched in, washed windows, scrubbed floors. Imagine all that furniture, all new at once: a new oil stove, new sofa in the kitchen and a new kitchen table with six chairs that even matched. There was new furniture in the parlor, new beds with real spring mattresses, bedside tables with lamps, and dressers, all brand new.

The local electrician came, removed the pennies from the fuse box, put in proper fuses and, for the first time in the history of the island, wall plugs were installed. But how to conceal the wiring for the chandelier in the parlor posed a problem. Several solutions were suggested but the best came from William Foote, a supposedly intellectually disabled man. He poked a hole in the ceiling where the chandelier was to go and stuffed in a fresh mackerel. He then cut a hole in the far corner of the room, pushed a young tomcat in with a string tied to its collar. The cat made its way to the mackerel and was brought down through the chandelier opening with the string and the wire attached.

The next highlight of the day came when the automatic washer and dryer were uncrated and carried in. Appropriate plumbing and electrical connections were made.

The ladies from the church organized refreshments: lobster sandwiches, homemade pies, cakes, candy, pop and coffee. This was a real party... a true island house warming. Outside of a furniture store, never before had anyone seen so much new stuff, and it all went into Arthur's house. His was the only house on the island with an indoor washer and dryer.

There was much rejoicing at his good fortune. Arthur gave away or burned all the old stuff and for the next three months, his wife was the envy of everyone in the village.

I saw Arthur every day, giving him moral support and whatever medication he needed for symptomatic relief. We had many interesting discussions and became very good friends. Arthur was a religious man, well adjusted and, having gone through the phases of denial and "why me?", he had done everything he could to prolong his life. He had had the best medical care possible and was accepting the inevitable result.

While I visited with him and his wife and their young daughter in their parlor the night before Arthur died, he reflected on his life as a fisherman, so dependent on the tides and storms of the Bay of Fundy, the size of the catch and the low price paid by the fish buyers. Arthur never had any money to spare but he did make a modest living, owned his house and his boat and had a happy family life.

That night, as we looked around his house with all that new furniture, he felt satisfied and philosophical.

"Doc," he told me, "in all my life I never had much money, but I done alright... and I finally beat those bastards in the finance company."

When Arthur died, the whole village turned out to remember and honour their own local hero, a brave and independent thinker who, facing a terrible dilemma with impossible odds stacked against him, made a courageous decision and won. If life were a baseball game, Arthur had hit a grand slam home run.

There is a biblical quotation often used at funerals: "When we are born we bring nothing into this world and we take nothing when we leave it." But this did not hold true for Arthur. Arthur, the independent thinker, an innovative leader who had made a fateful decision that astounded the entire community, brought nothing into this world when he was born, but when he left, he was a folk hero, a fighter, a legend in his own time, and he took six rooms of furniture... "all paid for by the damn finance company!"

CHAPTER FIVE
The Pentecostal Saga

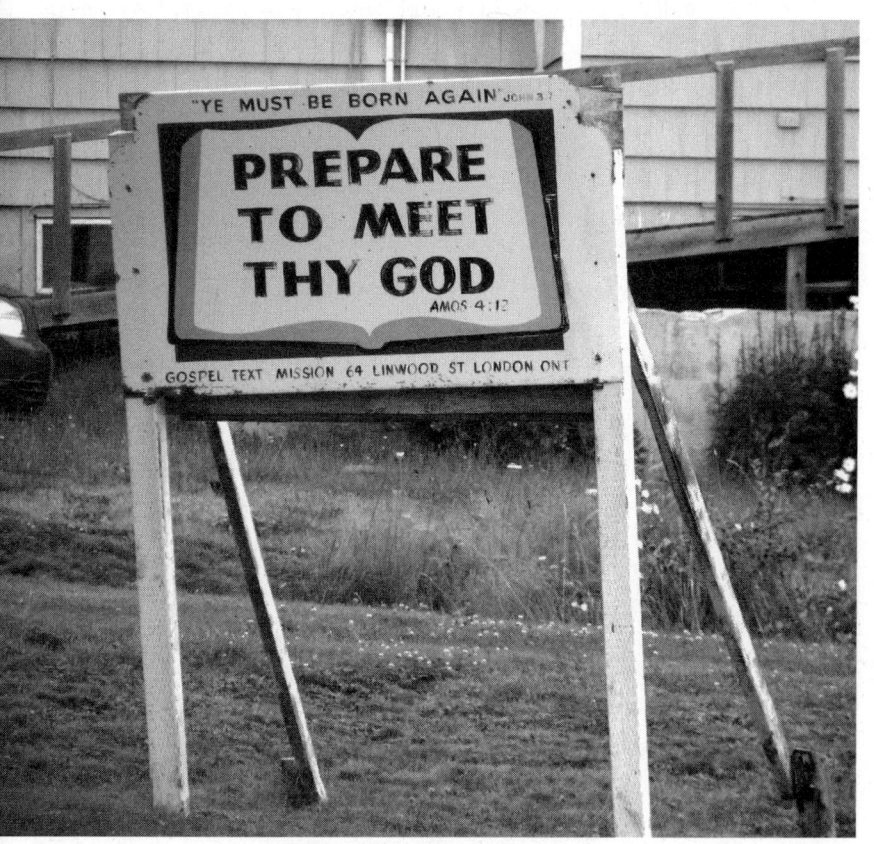

Two churches, one Baptist and the other a Pentecostal Tabernacle were located at Central Grove near the centre of our island. The tabernacle was a small wooden structure built by a group of dedicated people determined to convert and save the immortal souls of the islanders.

The building consisted of a small chapel sufficient to house about 50 worshippers. Crowded in were makeshift chairs, a small pulpit and several more chairs in front for the choir. Attached to the chapel were living quarters for the pastor and his family, consisting of his wife, daughter and son-in-law. Today we would describe the architecture as open concept – then, it was just that people could not afford partitions.

The number of parishioners grew. Services were held regularly and were well attended. I visited the family frequently, occasionally attending a church service, and also tending to medical needs, including the daughter's pregnancy. All was going smoothly.

The parson was a tall, no nonsense, dedicated man in his 50s, thin, balding and thoroughly convinced God had put him on earth to spread the Gospel. His wife, equally tall, a lean, serious lady with no makeup and steel-grey hair pulled tightly back into a small bun, was also dedicated and convinced of her husband's mission. Together, they resembled the classical picture of the Pennsylvania Dutch Quaker couple, standing forth, pitchfork in hand.

The parson was an interesting man. He had grown up in a poor family in the southern United States where he had worked as a farm labourer and was befriended by a preacher. He was recognized as a bright, potential scholar and entered a religious school, soon to become convinced that the Pentecostal Church was his calling. Through a variety of coincidences, he and his wife made their way to the Digby Islands, worked a small farm and built their church.

The reverend and I had some interesting talks. He was aware that I, as a Roman Catholic, would not be converted to his church. I found him a little too bombastic and threatening. I maintained that the God I knew was a more merciful, loving and forgiving creature, and that hell and damnation were not part of my final plan.

The parson's wife, I thought, was a more reasonable person, easier to talk to, a mother and about to become a grandmother for the first time. She was to be my assistant at the delivery of her daughter's child.

Preparations were made for the delivery well in advance. The baby's layette had been ordered from Eaton's catalogue and had arrived. I gave careful instruction in the use of four drops of chloroform. It was to be given for the relief of labour pains but only when specifically ordered by me. I was confident that everything was in order. Nothing could possibly go wrong. After all, I was the doctor.

My patient went into labour on a Sunday morning. I visited several times during the day. Elsie, via the EIN, and I were in constant contact; she was timing the pains. The whole village knew of the impending delivery.

A new drug called trilene had just become available for light anaesthesia and it was ideal for relief of early labour pain. It came in a container the size of a small flashlight and had a wrist strap so the woman could self-administer as she needed it. I had used it before and it worked well. Labour progressed and I expected the birth to be late afternoon or early evening.

Since it was Sunday, the parson was holding church service that evening. Needless to say, his wife, the only person in Central Grove who knew how to operate and play the pump organ, could not be at the service and she would be missed. Coincidentally, delivery of the baby was progressing at the same time as the Pentecostal service and the congregation knew it. Despite the parson's valiant efforts to preach religion, the congregation, almost all women, was more interested in what was going on in the next room, completely distracted as they listened for the sound of a baby's cry.

The delivery of a primipara is often more difficult. This one was no exception, taking a little longer and requiring several more drops of chloroform than usual. As the baby's head was delivered, I found the umbilical cord wrapped around the baby's neck. If too tight, it would cut off the baby's blood supply. I was able to unwrap the cord and the baby delivered, but was not breathing. I wiped its face, cleared mucous from its mouth, and gave it mouth-to-mouth resuscitation.

During the time I was concentrating on the baby, I was unaware that the entire congregation of 50 people had oozed through the door from the chapel into my case room. After a couple of my breaths into the babe, the little guy became pink and let out a loud and delightful cry. With that came another, much louder cry from the congregation: "And the Lord blew his breath into Moses... Halleluiah!"

The choir and the whole congregation – crowding into my case room, surrounding me, a new baby, and a hastily covered naked woman – burst into applause and sang their favourite hymns: *Christ is Risen, Jesus is Lord,* and *Let's All Gather at the River,* all loud enough for the entire village to hear.

I was on stage, albeit with a naked woman and a newborn baby, but I was a hero, a saint, a miracle worker, and I loved it. It was so uplifting I felt like a born-again Christian, a reformed sinner ready to give my testimony, even thinking there might be hope for my own salvation as I blurted out in unison with the congregation, "Thank you Jesus!"

The very serious, no nonsense parson joined in the celebration a happy man. It was the first time anyone had ever seen him laugh. The mother and baby thrived in a loving family, the parson and I became closer friends with better, mutual understanding. My very occasional attendance at one of his services gave him vain hope that there might be a conversion at hand but, hard as he tried, he was last heard to cry out in response to his failed efforts, "God, Oh God, why hast thou forsaken me?

Another "Pentecostal occasion" also involved a patient of mine, a 28-year-old mentally disabled, epileptic woman who was reasonably well controlled with medication under normal living conditions. She and her mother, who was also none too bright, came under the influence of the minister and were converted to the Pentecostal Church. Each gave testimony to the congregation. The mother's went well but the daughter, more than a little stressed, became excited as she was being "saved" and began yelling and screaming: "Jesus is Lord... I done bad things, runnin' the roads, makin' out wit the boys, and now I seen the light."

And with that, she went into an epileptic seizure. The shocked congregation rushed to gather round. The minister ordered, "Stand back, stand back, we'll pray." The mother hollered, "Pray my ass, give her them pills."

The girl recovered and the minister praised the Lord, pointing out that the seizure had been a sign, proving that God was in His heaven and now all was right with the world.

CHAPTER SIX
Eulalia (Granny) Tibert

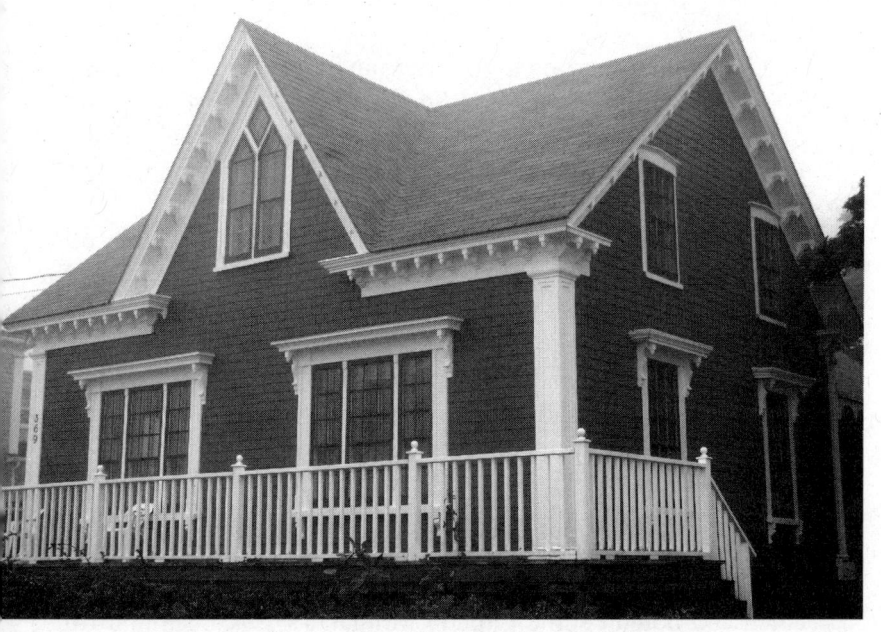

Long Island in Digby County is at the distal end of a 30-mile-long peninsula called Digby Neck. It separates the Bay of Fundy from St. Mary's Bay and the Acadian shore. Midway along Long Island is an area called Central Grove, which, in the early 50s, had several small farms and a lot of shoreline on both the Bay of Fundy on the north side and St. Mary's Bay on the south.

The matriarch of this area was Granny Tibert, an 85-year-old woman with severe angina pectoris. She was a tall, dignified, dominant and overweight religious hard-shell Baptist and past-president of the local chapter of the Nova Scotia Temperance Union.

Granny was married to Alvertus, an 87-year-old farmer/fisherman who still launched his 16-foot dory into the surf on the shore of St. Mary's Bay to tend to his lobster traps and catch whatever fish were running. He was a likeable, tough old guy and very tolerant of Eulalia.

Granny and Alvertus had a son, Earl, who, with three other men, earned a living long-line fishing and lobstering in both the Bay of Fundy and St. Mary's Bay. When they finished the day's catch they would go to the nearest fish buyer, either on the island or, if convenient, on the Acadian shore to sell their load. The Acadian shore was often preferred because a Nova Scotian government store there sold booze.

Our island was hard-shell Baptist and "dry". One morning, Earl came to my home/office with a black eye. He had obviously been in a fight, which he didn't remember. He said he had, with his partners, been to the French shore where they had sold their catch and bought some Captain Morgan's Black Diamond Rum, then, imbibing well, sailed home well after dark. When he woke up and saw his swollen, red and blackened eye, he went to his buddies, who assured him there had not been any fighting and that he had been alright when they left him the night before.

The story later unfolded that Earl's parents were in bed when he got home. He had kicked off his folded-down rubber boots and oilskins, lumbered up to bed and, with the help of Demerara medication, passed into dreamland.

Granny had heard Earl coming in and got up to investigate. She found him flat on his back, sound asleep and smelling of booze – right there, in her own home! She, who had been thoroughly schooled in the temperance movement and the horrors of demon rum, that threat to God-fearing people the world over, the cause of fornication, immorality, sin and social destruction, was overcome by a fit of righteous indignation and tough love. She closed her motherly fist and walloped Earl in the right eye.

In the 1950s, the management of angina pectoris consisted of bed rest, a nitroglycerine tablet placed under the tongue and, when necessary, morphine injected either subcutaneously or even intravenously. One or two newer drugs were available but not very helpful. I was called frequently to see Eulalia, usually at night. On at least two occasions, I could not hear a heartbeat, detect respiration or elicit reaction to painful stimulus. Then, as I was preparing to pronounce to the family that she was gone, Granny sat up and demanded a cup of tea.

The morphine injection, long before the convenient sterile injectable vials we have today, required a lighted candle to boil a teaspoonful of well water into which I dropped a quarter-grain morphine tablet. Then, with a 2-cc syringe, the now sterile morphine solution was withdrawn from the spoon and injected. The needles were reused and often barbed, but God was kind to this rural physician and no infection or other complication ever resulted.

I made daily visits, using more frequent and increasing doses of injectable morphine to supplement the nitroglycerine but Eulalia's angina continued and was becoming more and more severe. The situation was becoming desperate. I had to do something.

Having been raised in Cape Breton, and having had several ancestors who used Demerara black rum to treat any known and unknown disease, I wondered if Eulalia could possibly get some relief from her angina with alcohol. It was worth a try, but how was I to convince a life-long, tee totaling, "hard-shell" Baptist and local leader of the temperance union that there was some good to be derived from that horrible substance called alcohol? I was convinced that to stay alive, she needed it.

I crossed the ferry to the mainland and drove 30 miles to the nearest government store and bought two 40-ounce bottles of Bacardi White Rum. Then, with the help, advice and direction of my dietician wife, set about to disguise the offending substance. We poured 20-ounces into a 40-ounce, old style medicine bottle and added beet juice, chicken broth, vanilla, molasses, and a splash of Tabasco. We then fashioned a label claiming "newly discovered breakthrough in the treatment of angina pectoris." I gave this to Eulalia with instructions to shake well and take two ounces every three hours during the day and when needed at night.

The result was spectacular! For the first time in years, Granny Eulalia was without pain. She was able to resume activities as mother, grandmother and matriarch of the village. She could do a little gardening, go to church, play the organ and direct the choir. Eulalia became a local legend in the history of the hard-shell Baptist Church.

As the dedicated and fiery young pastor wound up his sermon on the evils of sin, dancing, fornication and alcohol, pleading "to let Jesus be your own personal saviour," Eulalia, as organist, choir director and the only card-carrying, tee totaling abolitionist member of the temperance society, herself drunk and hiccupping softly, led the congregation in rousing and uplifting renditions of *The Old Rugged Cross, Onward Christian Soldiers, Let's All Gather at the River* and lesser known come-all-yees like *She's Just a Piece of Driftwood a Drifting on the Sea, All She Needs is Jesus to No Longer Driftwood Be.*

Thanks to Granny Eulalia, the "prayer meetings" became more interesting and the talk of the island. They were the place to be and to be seen. The congregation grew and, with increasing popularity and public acclaim, Eulalia became more confident. She introduced newer toe-tapping and foot-stompin' hymns that shook the foundations of the little church. The hymns were similar to those of any southern Baptist community but islanders were assured they were certainly not Negro spirituals.

People came from the mainland and Brier Island to worship and pray at the Central Grove Baptist Church, which had to be enlarged. There was a corresponding marked increase in church collections, all due to Eulalia and demon rum.

The young pastor, obviously very happy with so many new converts attending, praying and worshipping in his church, could only say, "Thank you Jesus!"

Eulalia's medication kept me running back to the government store for more supplies and to the local grocer for the diluents. One morning, after weeks of refilling this special potion, Granny Eulalia's son, Earl, called to say his mother needed another bottle of medicine. I told him I had just delivered a bottle the night before. Earl, I knew, was a boozer and when he had come to realize that his mother's medicine made her feel good in ways very similar to some of his own experiences, he became suspicious and decided he should sample the "wonderful breakthrough" in the treatment of coronary artery disease.

When Earl called me, he asked, "That medicine's for her heart, ain't it?" Without waiting for a reply, he went on, "Well, I've got a hellova bad heart too."

He had discovered the main ingredient of my secret formula. My secret was blown... and Eulalia was outraged. She accused me of being an infidel, even an antichrist. She became so worked up she had a severe angina attack. The pain was so bad, morphine and nitroglycerine were not sufficient to provide relief. Much to her own consternation, Eulalia's only recourse was a double dose of my special medicine. And it worked! Pain is a powerful persuader.

After cooling down, and with the pain relieved, she agreed to continue with my special formula but only on the condition of sworn and absolute confidentiality. No one else in the village, the Digby Islands, the church or the temperance society could ever know that she was a closet alcoholic.

Eulalia continued for three years on her medication and I have often reflected on the interesting conflict between the lone young country doctor, pledged to save and/or prolong every life, and the older, highly principled religious zealot equally determined to live and even die for the strong beliefs on which she had built her life. Was I justified in giving a patient medication that I knew was in violation of her rights, even though it saved her life, made her comfortable and a productive member of society?

Realizing that Eulalia had lived for years with angina before I met her, it is possible that she might have continued with her pain without my medication, but she did become more comfortable with its use and I was convinced she lived longer because of it.

She was also better able to contribute to the community. She brought more people into her church, people who came to recognize that there was a God, a life hereafter, and that all should lead decent and moral lives. This would not have happened had the young country doctor, attempting to follow the dictates of the Hippocratic Oath and the fundamental principle, "First do no harm," not fraudulently tricked a loyal, God fearing, life-long, aggressive teetotaler and trusting patient into becoming an alcoholic.

Eulalia's secret has been kept for 50 years. If there is a statute of limitations, it is now passed and the vault can be opened and the story told.

The philosopher Thomas Aquinas taught that the end does not justify the means. I have often wondered, if that most learned and respected thinker had been a young, inexperienced country doctor, alone on an island facing an impossible contradiction, might he have allowed just one exception to his rule?

CHAPTER SEVEN
The Bloody Big Snow Storm

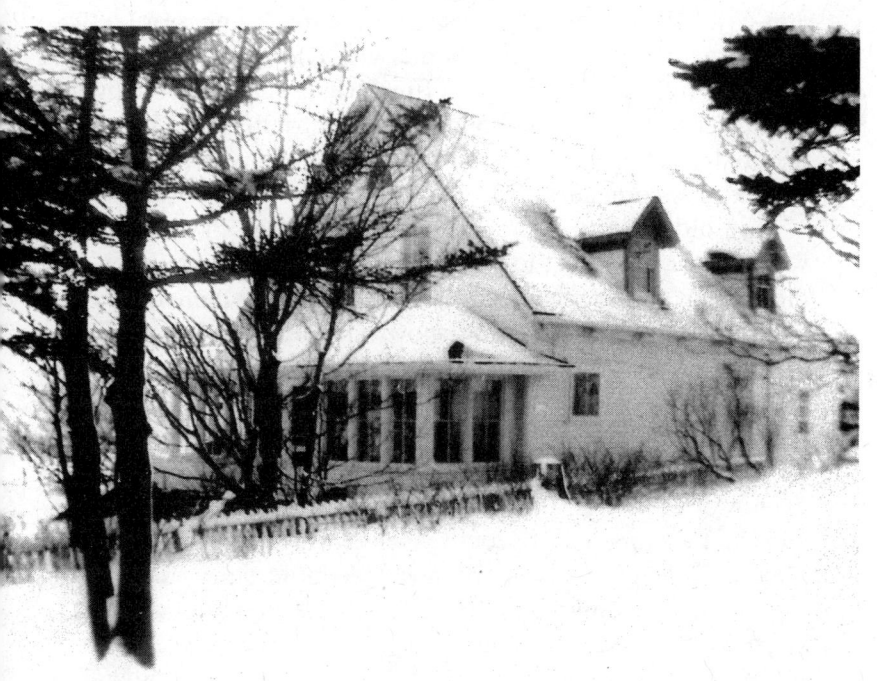

Life for us on Long Island was very comfortable. When home renovations were complete, we had a new furnace, a new kitchen, a fireplace, decoration, and Katie's parents' old but beautiful furniture. We had, by island standards, a luxurious house, a new baby, and the thrill of being a country doctor with a family and the respect and trust of the community. Life couldn't possibly be better.

The island, sticking out into the Bay of Fundy, was subject to occasional violent storms, including heavy snow falls lasting several days. During these storms, with the roads impassable, I had no alternative but to stay at home with Katie and play with our two-year-old son in front of the fireplace, or read with the light of a kerosene lamp while hoping the electricity would soon be restored, trusting there would be no need for my medical services until the storm subsided.

The old country doctors used to boast that, "If you can get word to me, I will get to you, my patient." That was fine before the days of the telephone and ham radio but on the island, blanketed by two to three feet of snow whipped into large drifts by howling winds, any travel was nigh impossible, yet getting word to me had become relatively easy.

As one of these big storms abated, and before the road could be cleared or the electricity restored, we settled in for a quiet evening in front of a wood fire. Katie was three months pregnant and feeling a little rocky. Our two-year-old was a happy, playful little guy. I read the usual bedtime story, tucked him into bed, came downstairs and looked at the outside world. The storm had blown over, leaving a beautiful winter scene with a full moon glistening on the pristine, newly fallen snow and the church steeple. God was in his heaven and all was right with the world.

About ten o'clock, Katie decided to turn in. I wanted to read a little while longer but within minutes I heard her cry out. She had made it upstairs but, without warning, had begun to bleed profusely; she was having a miscarriage. I ran upstairs, helped her into bed and immediately realized the need for a D & C... and the impossibility of getting her to the hospital in Digby 40 miles and a ferry ride away. The only alternative I had in order to slow or stem the hemorrhaging was to do a vaginal packing.

I ran downstairs to the office where I had the necessary sterile supplies and equipment, put them on a tray and ran back upstairs. Katie had gotten out of bed, still bleeding heavily, and fallen to the floor. As I ran into the room, I slid on the blood on the hardwood floor and fell on top of her, spilling my sterile supplies everywhere.

I gathered myself and lifted Katie back into bed. The most beautiful woman in the world and the only one I had ever loved, the mother of my only son, was bleeding to death in my arms and I, the cocky young doctor who knew everything, could do nothing about it. In a moment of inspiration and desperation, I called Elsie.

"I need help," I cried, and told her that Katie was bleeding uncontrollably and had to get to the hospital. The all-knowing Elsie, cool and capable under pressure, said Clyde Stark had a big truck. He could probably get through. She called him, told him the doctor's wife was having a miscarriage and had to get to the hospital, and that he had to help.

"What's a miscarriage?" was Clyde's response.

"No time for explanations," Elsie said. "Just get your truck and break a path from the doctor's house to the ferry."

"Jesus, the road is covered wit tree feet a snow!" Clyde argued.

"I know the road is blocked!" Elsie told him. "Just get your damn truck out Clyde, and break a path for the doctor."

"Okay, anything for the doc."

Clyde was five miles away but within half an hour he was standing in my kitchen with the big truck purring in the driveway. At that point, every soul on the island, listening on the party line, knew everything. Needless to say, this was long before the current privacy laws.

Gene Tibert, our next door neighbour, hollered at me from downstairs. Elsie had called him too. He was a big strong young man and, with Katie wrapped in blankets, carried her downstairs, through the living room, the dining room and into the kitchen, ready to go out the door to the truck.

Katie, prostrate, was conscious when lying down but passed

out if she sat up. There was not enough room in the cab of the truck for her to lie down so Clyde suggested he chain my 1952 Chevy to the back of the truck and tow us along. He backed the big flatbed up to the front of the Chevy. With heavy chains around the front axel of the car and the big iron bars of the truck, there was not an inch between the two vehicles. One headlight got broken and the radiator grill was caved in during the hookup.

"Sorry about that," Clyde muttered, "...but let's go!"

Gene had started the car to warm it up, carried Katie out and laid her on the back seat of the car. I sat on the floor holding her and, with Gene in the driver's seat, Clyde gunned the big truck and the Chevy crunched, scraped and banged into the big iron bars at the back of the flatbed. The radiator was completely destroyed but Clyde kept us going, beating our way through the island's 10 miles to the ferry.

Thinking ahead once again, Elsie had alerted the ferrymen to be waiting and watching for us. There was a full moon so the tide was high around midnight. The ferry boat was, therefore, at the top of the ramp. I was amazed at the graceful way a seasoned fisherman could dance his way from the slippery seaweed-covered ramp to a shifting boat without stumbling or missing a step. He didn't even seem to have to look where he was going... and he was carrying my Katie.

With the Bay of Fundy tide running through the narrow Petite Passage, the ferry had to run along the shore 300-400 yards against the tide. As it started to cross, it was swept downstream and had to creep the 300-400 yards along the opposite shore to get to the dock.

Elsie had arranged for a car to meet us on the mainland side. She had even, in the middle of the night, persuaded the Nova Scotia Department of Highways to have a monster snowplow clear the road for us. I never knew how she managed that but as some island philosopher told me later: "That don't surprise me none; nobody don't f...k with Elsie."

On reaching the other side, Gene once again carried Katie to the waiting warm car, engine running. With her lying on the back seat, me on the floor, and Gene at the wheel, we followed the snowplow. This part of the trip took another hour, which seemed to go on forever.

Elsie had called the hospital so when we arrived Katie was rushed into the operating room. In a rural hospital, emergencies are treated as emergencies. No time is wasted with administration, documentation, identification or paperwork. Everyone knows everybody anyway. The attitude is, "Let's get the job done and do the incidentals later."

Dr. John McCleave, a mountain of a man at well over six-foot-three, and probably 300 pounds, was a most skillful surgeon. He was big, confident and likeable, and he was waiting for us. Katie's hemoglobin level was down to 15 percent of normal. She was now unconscious. Fortunately, the Digby Blood Bank was in the hospital. Katie's blood was taken for typing and cross matching. Dr. McCleave ordered four units of Type O, RH Negative to be started immediately while he did the D & C to save her life.

In the recovery room, four more bottles of blood arrived in glass containers resembling elongated Classic Coca Cola bottles. Each had a rubber stopper through which was inserted a large bore trocar. Rubber tubing with an in-line mesh filter was attached to that. Frequently, the filter clogged and had to be cleared or replaced, hopefully maintaining a semblance of sterility in the process.

I sat with Katie all night, monitoring the transfusions and re-starting them each time the filter clogged. By daylight, she had recovered from the anaesthetic and regained consciousness. God was back in His heaven and we mortals began to breathe easier – until I had a moment of panic. I remembered that in the emergency, I had forgotten our two-year-old at home. I called Elsie (who else) and told her and she assured me that all was well with our child. Shirley, our next door neighbour (Gene's wife) had taken our son to her house where he was playing happily with her two-year-old. Then I also told Elsie that, thanks to her, Katie was out of danger. My world was beginning to recover.

One of the hospital nurses provided me with a scrub suit and took my blood-soaked clothes home, washed, ironed and returned them. My 1952 Chevy, with the front end wrecked and the motor seized, had been towed into the dealership by Clyde and declared a write-off. Coincidentally, but not surprisingly, the dealer had a new one waiting for me.

With Katie now stable and out of danger, but being kept in hospital for another few days, I returned to the island. To my great surprise, the bloody mess I had left in the bedroom and the trail of blood down the stairs, through the living room, kitchen and out the door, was nowhere to be seen. The house was immaculate. The women of the village had invaded. They cleaned, scrubbed, vacuumed and polished. The house had never been so clean; not a trace of the disaster I had left the night before remained.

I was then treated to a magnificent lobster dinner. Katie's homecoming was also a special event. The ladies of the village brought food: cakes, pies, home-canned goods and a whole lot of other stuff. The men brought lobsters, scallops and fresh fish.

When Clyde Stark came to visit, we could hardly express enough gratitude. This had to be the best place in the world to live. As Katie regained strength she had to deal with the involuntary depression that invariably follows a miscarriage and the loss of a wanted pregnancy. The sense of inadequacy, guilt, anger, and why-me can be overwhelming.

"Couldn't I have done something to keep this from happening?" she asked herself. "It must have been my fault."

The problem is exacerbated by the severe blood loss, fatigue, and the realization of having been through a life-threatening experience.

However, in a shorter time than most women, Katie not only recovered but was also better than ever despite, or perhaps because of what had happened. Her recovery was sped up when the local home and school association was persuaded by the Nova Scotia Department of Education to do some local community activity, like putting on a play. The play suggested was the story of an Irish princess who was reported to be travelling incognito in Canada. Katie, with her Irish heritage, was the only one in town who could do an Irish accent and naturally became, not only the lead actress, but also the director and producer of a play called *Princess O'Toole*. And that, my friends, is an entirely different story.

CHAPTER EIGHT
Princess O'Toole

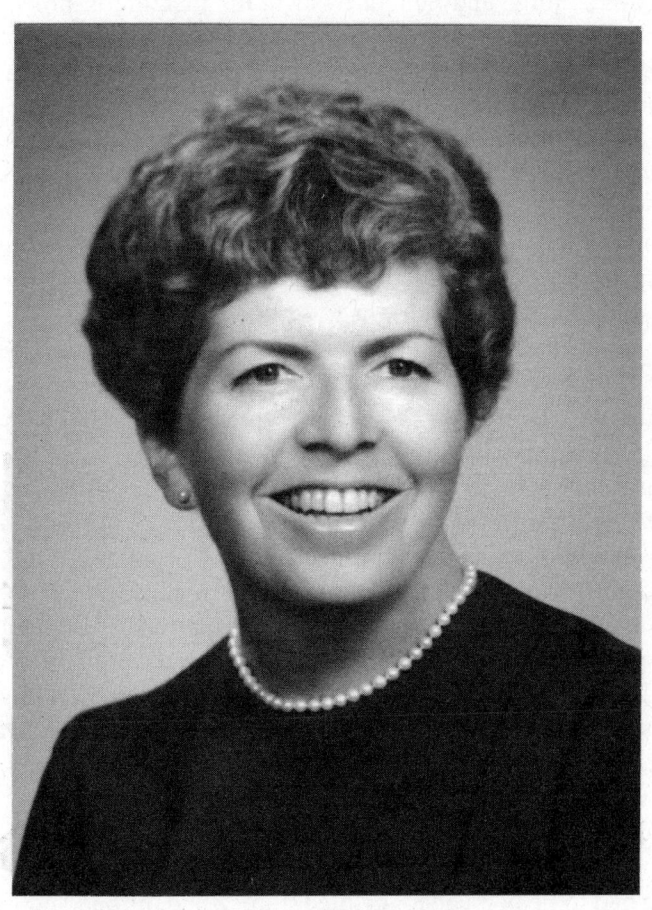

With the advent of television in the early 50s, the Nova Scotia Department of Education and the social services department felt rural communities would need activities to compete with, or even counteract the effects of the new "electronic influence". They hit upon a plan whereby rural villages, such as Freeport, might be persuaded to do something to stimulate community spirit and co-operation. With this policy in place, the Department of Education dispatched a representative to speak to a Home and School Association meeting in Freeport.

An attempt was already being made to amalgamate the three one-room rural schools on the island but it was encountering considerable resistance. Those who "came from away", including two people from a sociological research team from Cornell University, held the predictable position that a school with separate rooms for each grade would be better than one with 12 grades in one room, taught by one lonely teacher. The opposite view was easily summed up by the often heard local statement: "I went to that school and I done alright."

The Cornell researchers cautioned us to be patient because "social change takes time." Other than that, Home-and-School discussions focused on the weighty question: "What do we have for the next meeting, doughnuts or sandwiches?"

Into this parochial world, the representative of the education department came to urge the ladies of the Home and School Association to organize a drama group to wile away the long winter nights. He produced six copies of a play called Princess O'Toole. The story was about a penniless, dirt poor Irish girl who came to Canada with charm and beauty but bereft of material goods. At the same time, it was rumored that a wealthy Irish princess was travelling in the country incognito. Needless to say, there was confusion and the penniless little lady was mistaken for the wealthy princess and, therefore, treated as royalty.

The cast of characters consisted of four men and four women but only one man in the village fancied himself an actor; the other three had to be persuaded, cajoled, threatened, bribed and bullied, but they finally agreed.

The four women were a much easier sell, particularly since the doctor's wife, with a strong Irish heritage and a lust for the theatre with all its fame and adulation, leaped at and seized the opportunity to play the lead role... and led the charge to enroll three more women.

Katie quickly became the organizer, director, producer, costume designer, stage manager and general factotum for the entire enterprise. Parts were assigned, the script memorized and rehearsals went on all winter. No other activity in the village held a candle to the upcoming theatrical blockbuster. Princess O'Toole had everything and was everything. The village held its collective breath.

Two of the most interested observers, of course, were the Cornell researchers, a husband and wife team with whom Kate and I became good friends. They were keenly interested in the project from the sociological point of view... just how, or if, this would engage the community, but also because of their personal contact with Katie, the theatre impresario, and her efforts to keep the cast focused, arrange rehearsal times, and co-ordinate all with the tides to accommodate fishermen's schedules – not to mention the necessity of negotiating personnel and ego challenges that became public with such outbursts as, "She's got better lines than me."

Rehearsals were held in parlors previously used only for funerals and weddings and in the Baptist Church hall. They seemed to go on forever but finally, after a long winter, opening night approached. Notices were put up in the post office in each village, and in three village general stores. It was even announced during church services the Sunday before. Excitement grew. Nothing like this had ever been done before. Sure, there had been travelling performances staged in the village, but this was local talent.

An outside group called The Epley Sisters, a seven-girl musical troupe from the southern states, had visited the year before. They were billed as a religious revival group and they whooped it up with every known musical instrument. Their hit number was *The Old Rugged Cross,* and if you ever heard their rendition, played with bugle, slide trombone, tenor sax and drums, with a

Beatles kind of beat, you would never again be satisfied with the conventional version.

Katie and I had attended the seven sisters' concert in the Baptist Church and when we, two Roman Catholics, entered, we were greeted like the proverbial prodigal children returning to the fold and were ushered up to the front pew. When The Epley Sisters reached their crescendo and hollered, "Do you want Jesus Christ to be your own personal saviour?" I had to restrain my Katie. My convent-bred and previously thoroughly brain washed Irish Roman Catholic wife, caught up in the excitement, in an uncharacteristic explosion of religious fervor, was damn near a born-again Christian.

The cast survived the ordeal of a winter of rehearsals for Princess O'Toole and opening night finally came. The stage was set. The crowd of souls from three villages filled the church hall. The energy was palpable, the tension high.

Twenty minutes before curtain time, I was sitting with the Cornell couple when Katie summoned me. There was an unanticipated crisis. The four male actors, all big, strong, able-bodied fishermen, afraid of absolutely nothing heretofore, men who faced life-threatening situations in the Bay Of Fundy every day of their lives, were struck with stage fright and collectively refused to go on. What was Katie to do? The situation called for a means of instilling courage into these brave men.

As a native Cape Bretoner, I recalled the old Scottish proverb of the little grey mouse in Glasgow, which, upon licking spilled whiskey off the bar, stood on its hind legs, thumped its chest and hollered: "Now bring on your gawddamn cat."

I had the necessary supplies in the trunk of my car, normally used only as treatment for snake bite, occasionally for temporary anaesthesia while removing a fish hook embedded in a fisherman's hand, and often as an inducement when I had to ask a favour of an islander. I had never met an island man who refused a drink... as long as his wife was not in view.

The four men, now cowering in a back room of the Baptist Church hall, afraid of nothing in the world except of appearing on stage in front of the whole community, were easily enticed outside to the trunk of my car where I happened to have a 40-ouncer of black rum and another of Johnnie Walker Scotch. I opened the bottles and passed them around. Relaxation was immediate. With the bottles quickly drained and courage restored, the guys bravely marched back into the hall, willing and anxious to emulate the acting skills of John Barrymore.

But another problem then surfaced. Katie immediately sensed what I had done and, while not entirely in agreement with the treatment administered for stage fright, she thought that if it worked, maybe the play could go on. The other three women, all strict temperance addicts, had a distinctly different reaction. They became enraged at the male players, now showing increasing signs of inebriation, and stormed off the stage and out the door.

Katie, attempting to rescue the performance she had worked so hard to produce, pleaded with the women, but alcohol had been consumed very near to the back hall of their Baptist Church. That disgrace could never be tolerated. What would people think? "We're out of here!" was their common cry. And they would not come back.

On her own Katie set up four chairs on the stage for the male actors, who, by this time were blind drunk and absolutely inarticulate. The curtain parted, the applause rang out. The men, not knowing where they were and almost falling off their chairs, gave the performance of their lives.

Katie, absolute mistress of the situation, adroitly smoothed out the rough parts, reciting much of the play with narrative transitions such as: "As Sean would say, if he were able...," and she would then quote from the script. Then, "As Rory would say, if he were able..." Or, "As Kathleen might say, if she were here... And Princess O'Toole would say..." The Cornell researchers were impressed with the performance and asked later if that was really the way the production had been planned.

After the opening night performance, a crowd gathered at our house with champagne, just as they do on Broadway, and anxiously awaited the critics' reviews. Since there were no overnight newspapers on the island, more time was required.

Someone recalled that classic exchange between Winston

Churchill and George Bernard Shaw in which Shaw sent two tickets to Churchill for one of his opening performances, along with a note saying, "Bring a friend, if you have one." Churchill replied," I can't make it opening night, but I can attend a second performance, if there is one."

Regrettably, there was never a second performance of Princess O'Toole. The critics eventually surfaced... divided along gender lines. The ladies' quilting circle, composed of strict temperance followers, was very negative because alcohol had been consumed and, at that, so close to the church! The women in the play had done the right thing by storming out, and whoever was responsible should be ashamed.

Male opinions were divided. Those who gathered around the post office waiting for the bus and arrival of the daily mail seemed indifferent. In the general store, the crowd traditionally gathered around the sauerkraut barrel, which was seen as the most accurate and reliable, if primitive, barometer and predictor of weather. With increased barometric pressure, the sauerkraut was pressed below the surface of the vinegar. This meant good weather for fishing. This group had a different take on Princess O'Toole. They spoke as one man. If given the opportunity to get a skinful of free booze, whether behind the Baptist Church, in front of it, or anywhere else, they'd go for it. If their wives happened to object, and they would, they'd eventually get over it. The community-wide pro-and-con discussion went on for days and weeks.

Katie became known as the Princess of O'Toole. The village men wanted to do another production and, strangely, numerous applications for male parts in the cast came forward. But, alas, the women ruled and vowed never again. Dramatic efforts on Long Island, Digby County, came to an ignominious and inglorious end.

CHAPTER NINE

The Second Big Snow Storm

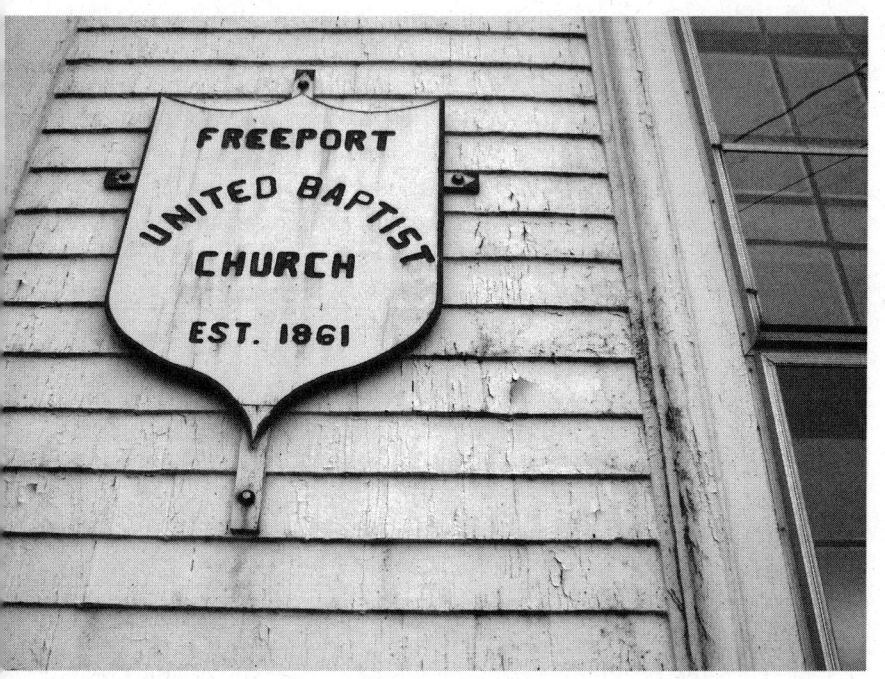

The blizzard of 1954 was not unexpected, and was one of the worst in recent memory. The island was again covered in two to three feet of snow with big drifts and howling winds. I recalled the frightening situation of the year before when, under similar circumstances, I had to get Katie to the hospital. This time, as I sat once again storm-stayed before my fireplace with my family in absolute comfort and safety, I was hoping and praying that no medical emergency would arise.

The island road was tended by Clyde Stark, the same man who engineered the rescue of my family the year before. In the interim, the government had supplied him with a small caterpillar tractor to scrape the gravel road in summer. For winter, a wooden cab was built on and a snowplow blade attached.

When this storm hit, Clyde, with his trusty little tractor, determined the road had to be cleared before another crisis developed. With his Lindberg cap and its dangling, flapping ear lugs, a heavy old torn and stained army great coat with some of the original brass buttons still attached, heavy woolen pants, Stanfield long red underwear, big lumberman boots and heavy lobster mitts, Clyde started in Tiverton and ploughed through 10 miles of snow drifts to Freeport.

The tractor, a rusty old derelict, had seen most of its life on the mainland and now, in semi-retirement, was relegated to the island. Among his other talents, Clyde was what the islanders called a good "dirty-hand mechanic" and as such, was able to keep the old tractor in a semblance of running order. Spare parts were never available so he jury-rigged, chicken-wired, cannibalized and stole parts from any number of old trucks, retired fishing boat engines and shipwrecks.

The only problem he could not remedy was the engine coil, an electrical device contained in a small black cylinder about the size of a flashlight and attached to the engine with four bolts. It had a heavy wire leading in and several smaller wires coming out. Inside, electrical "stuff" was immersed in oil. This item is crucial to the operation of the internal combustion engine. A problem arises when the oil inside the coil gets too cold, becomes too viscid and shuts down the engine.

Having frequently had that experience with the old tractor, and having begged, borrowed and, yes, even stolen coils from other sources, the problem persisted but Clyde, as we learned, was able to cope with this and any other situation. His solution was surprisingly simple. Whenever the engine quit, which was usually in a snowdrift and under heavy load, Clyde would unbolt the coil and take it to the nearest house. Houses on the island were never locked and the oil stove in the kitchen was always on. It was often the only means of heating a house. Clyde could go into any house, put his coil in the oven, make himself a pot of tea, sit down and wait for the coil to warm up. Sometimes the sleeping residents never knew he had ever been there. Everyone knew and trusted Clyde and was delighted to be able to help him on his way.

When the coil was heated and dry, Clyde would return to the snowbound tractor, bolt the coil onto the engine, connect the wires and continue the ploughing job. As one poetic islander described his efforts:

"As the engine varoomed, spluttered and died,
'twas the coil, Clyde knew, it had died.
So off it came, and out he went
Into the snow, the wind and the din
In search of a stove in a house,
That would let him in."

Throughout that long and stormy night, Clyde visited numerous houses with his disabled coil, got it defrosted each time, bolted it back onto the engine and continued on his way. His goal had been to make his way across the island as far as the doctor's house where, although having reached his destination, he once again found himself stalled in a snowdrift, this time equidistant from my house and the nearby Baptist Church.

He appeared in my kitchen clutching his trusty coil in his lobster mitt, looking tired, frozen cold, disheveled and forlorn. I took the coil from him, put it in the oven, peeled off his great coat and sat him beside the open oven door to thaw out. He had been on the tractor since 4 o'clock the afternoon before and was starving.

Katie loaded him up with bacon and eggs, toast and coffee. I offered Demerara black rum and he took a good double. When the coil was dry and Clyde defrosted, he thanked us for the food and hospitality, took his coil, secured it with the four bolts, connected the wires and started the engine.

Clyde Stark was a big, strong, powerful man and independent thinker. He did not join the Masons or the Independent Order of Foresters Lodge at the time. He did not go to church and was reported to have liked strong drink, a characteristic not favoured by the hard-shell Baptist community. Katie and I watched in amazement as he, with a hitherto unknown hostility toward the Baptist way of life, now fueled by rum supplied by the Roman Catholic doctor, turned his tractor 90 degrees to the left and headed straight for the Baptist Church, ploughed through the front yard, up the steps and shattered the big oak double doors.

Fortunately, the tractor got stuck in the door jamb and stalled. Katie and I ran over, pulled the semi-inebriated Clyde out of it and brought him back to our house.

It was later discovered by the Baptist community that the demon rum that had caused the shattering of the doors and almost destroyed the rest of their church had been prescribed and administered by the Roman Catholic doctor.

In fear and trembling, Clyde went into hiding to wait for the predictable ecclesiastical wrath to die down. Such wrath would have been reasonable, given the hostile relationship that had existed between the community and the belligerent Irish Catholic Doctor Hugh O'Reilly, who had lived on the island for a short time before Katie and I arrived. He had been asked to take part in a November 11th memorial day ceremony at the cenotaph in front of the Baptist Church and his response, unreasonable, curt, obnoxious and shocking, was: "I'll not set foot on yer gawddamn Baptist Church grounds."

I had heard this story and feared there might be a negative reaction to me after the church door incident. It never happened.

In the Roman Church, priests committed to doing missionary work around the world followed a number of orders, such as to teach and spread Roman Catholic doctrine wherever possible.

When Katie and I decided to settle in Freeport, we visited the local parish priest in Digby. He was a rather large, obese, aggressive, over confident Irish Bostonian, at the time serving temporarily at the small parish between assignments in Peru and God knew where else. He told us he was a missionary of the Oblate Order and, among other things, welcomed our going to Freeport.

He had heard that several Catholic families who had settled on the islands were now "fallen away from the true church" because of the distance and, worse still, were "in danger of becoming Baptist."

Father Dermot Murphy thought Katie and I were a whole lot more devout than we really were and we figured this man, the modern version of a missionary, was a whole lot less dedicated than the original Canadian Martyrs. He suggested he could use us as a wedge to spread the gospel to the Digby Islands and he, or one of his fellow Irish Bostonian priests, would come to Freeport to say mass at our house. All we had to do was round up the 12 or 15 lost souls, invite them to mass, pick them up at the Westport ferry dock, meet the priest at the Tiverton ferry dock 10 miles away, bring them all to our house, feed them brunch and help save their immortal souls.

Coincidentally, the day the repair work on the Baptist Church doors was completed, Father Murphy called to announce he would come to Freeport the following Sunday to say mass in our house, and would we please assemble the flock.

As we all knew, there were no secrets on the island; all calls were monitored by Elsie. In no time, the whole village knew of the impending visit of a Catholic priest. The reaction was swift.

Elsie called to say, "You don't have enough chairs in your house for 15 people. We'll bring some across the road from our church."

So, on the first Sunday of having Catholic mass celebrated on the island, we had 15 forgotten Catholic bums on Baptist chairs. All worshipping, undoubtedly, the same God! This was obviously the way ecumenism should work.

In time, the Baptist minister announced he was leaving Freeport. The church had advertised for a replacement and had five applications from men of varying qualifications, two were divinity school graduates, one a previous lay reader, one had received a call from the Lord while carrying a carcass in a meat packing factory, and one just wanted to try it.

The church authorities had some difficulty interpreting the resumes and, in desperation, or wisdom, came in a delegation to Katie and me, two Roman Catholics, to aid them in choosing their new Baptist minister. We were able to shorten the list to two applicants and finally chose one, with whom Katie and I eventually became very good friends. We had a very happy association and agreed bigotry did not exist in our small world.

The memory of Clyde Stark as a special friend – how he saved Katie's life and how he and I together nearly wrecked the Baptist Church – is deeply ingrained in our minds.

We were saddened to learn of his death in 1963 but overjoyed when, in 2008, more than 50 years since we left Freeport, we met Clyde's son, Rodney. I remembered Rodney, his brother and two sisters as kids but had lost track of the family when Katie and I moved to Halifax. I asked Rodney what he had been doing since the last time I saw him and this was his reply:

"I was born in the Digby General Hospital on January 13, 1947. In 1949, the family moved to Freeport where we operated a small sheep farm. I attended all three Island schools. I left home in 1961 to work with my father at J. D. Irving Marine on tug boats on the Saint John River. Originally employed there as a second class engineer, I was later promoted to chief engineer.

"I returned to Freeport in late 1965 and have worn many hats since then: millwright, oil agent, furnace repairer and installer, ambulance operator and paramedic for 18 years (with W. A. MacIntyre and then with Digby County Ambulance as manager and operator, Freeport Area). I was also employed as a fisherman, machinist, and then in refrigeration and diesel repair.

"An on-the-job injury forced me to leave the workforce in April, 1989. After a few years of recovery I became interested in acrylic painting. I am now a self-taught artist and do very

detailed works of nautical themes, landscapes and local histori-cally based pictures.

"I still live in Freeport with my wife, Leta. We have grown children and both of us work in stained glass. A few years ago we purchased an antique car that we enjoy working on together and traveling in around the province. "

I saw some of Rodney's work and was most impressed with his acrylic painting of the "Shipwreck", a beautiful picture of a full-rigged barque run aground in rough seas. I have the original in my collection, reproduced in this book.

CHAPTER TEN

All I ever Knew About Psychiatry

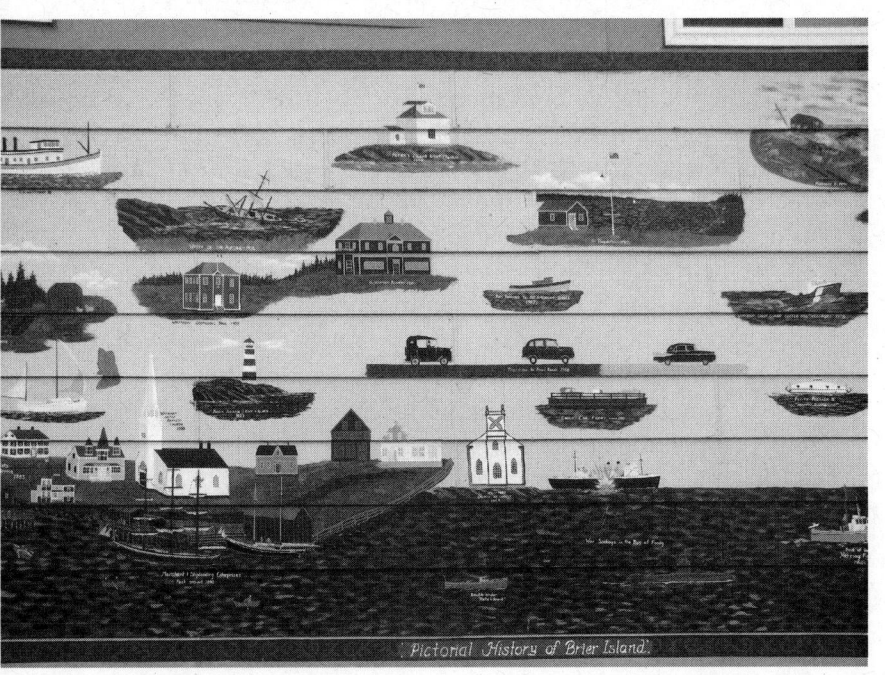

Pictorial History of Brier Island

All I ever new about psychiatry I learned from a Newfoundlander on a quiet moonlit night in Freeport – Freeport was always quiet at night, but not often moonlit. The silence of that particular night was shattered by a number of blasts from a double-barreled, 12-gauge shotgun. Startled villagers peeked out through curtained windows and from between barely opened doors as half a dozen brave men assembled around Connors' Store and the local one-room post office. The trigger happy culprit was found: a well known village loner, a depressed, sad-sack little man with no family. He lived alone, worked part time as an unskilled labourer and took no part in community activities. He didn't even go to Saturday night movies at the Baptist Church.

But until that moonlit night, this guy had never been in trouble with the law. To the village he was just "poor little Archie": pitied, tolerated, not disliked and never feared. It must have been the full moon and the demons that came out that night – Archie flipped or, as a local mechanic put it, "He blew a gasket!"

He had loaded up his old 12-guage, taken a handful of shells from the top shelf of his kitchen cupboard and decided to show other people that he too was really somebody. He walked down the road toward Connors' Store – the village centre – blasting off his shotgun into the night air, hurting no one and damaging nothing, just making noise and muttering incoherently.

In times of emergency like this the local volunteer constabulary, consisting of anyone brave enough to venture out, swung into action. The doctor was often called to give the offender "a shot" to quiet him down but Archie was a very passive guy and gave up the shotgun without argument. He didn't need the shot from the doctor, he just wanted to talk to someone who would listen and not find fault. So who else but the patient, friendly and likeable country doctor got the opportunity to spend the night with Archie? The others went home to bed.

Archie was lonely; he had no friends and thought no one liked him. He was a loser, a Grade 6 dropout. Life was just not worth living. He and I talked all night and by morning I was able to convince him that there was help available through psychiatric services at the Sick Mariners' Hospital. Needless to say, the service was only for mariners, including fishermen, and Archie was neither a mariner nor a fisherman. But by some mysterious coincidence, he was notified that he was a registered deckhand on a big fishing boat and thus qualified to go to Mariners' Hospital, part of Camp Hill Hospital in Halifax. I never knew how that came about but I did make the arrangements, found a reason to go to Halifax and took Archie with me.

The world being small... and smaller yet in Nova Scotia, I was delighted to discover the psychiatrist assigned to look after Archie was Edward O'Brian Freeman, a classmate of mine at St. Francis Xavier University. He was a Newfoundlander, had gone to medical school in Ireland, and was now a third-year resident in psychiatry at Camp Hill.

I hadn't seen my old friend for years and was happy to link up with him again. Dr. Edward O'Brian Freeman was easy going, relaxed, likeable – a lovable Newfoundlander – as most "Newfies" are. He made Archie feel welcome in the hospital.

About three weeks later, I had occasion to go to Halifax and went to see my old friend and check on how Archie was doing. Edward told me he was doing fine, that he was friendly, cooperative and fitting into the hospital routine... but there was one problem. As Edward put it, "He seems sad all the time."

I told Ed that I had known Archie at least three years. He had always been a sad sack, very much like a long ago L'il Abner comic strip character called Mr. Pfffith, a little guy who was always under a black cloud. It rained everywhere he went. Archie had shown no variation in this type of behaviour until that moonlit night when he shot up the village.

Ed reflected on that and, in classic Newfie wisdom, cutting through the jargon, psychobabble and doublespeak, he summed up for me the essence of psychiatry in one sentence: "I think we've cured his psychosis, but we're stuck with his personality."

After a month or two with Dr. Freeman, Archie returned to the island, clean shaven and neatly dressed, a different man from the one who had left under such a black cloud. He held his head high and his chest out and he walked with a new air of confidence. Doctor Freeman had worked a miracle.

Archie was able to get a job at Connors' Fish Plant and became friendly, worked steadily, and lived a happier life – without psychosis. He was welcomed back into the village and never again missed the western movies at the Baptist Church hall.

CHAPTER ELEVEN

A Day in the Life
of a Country Doctor

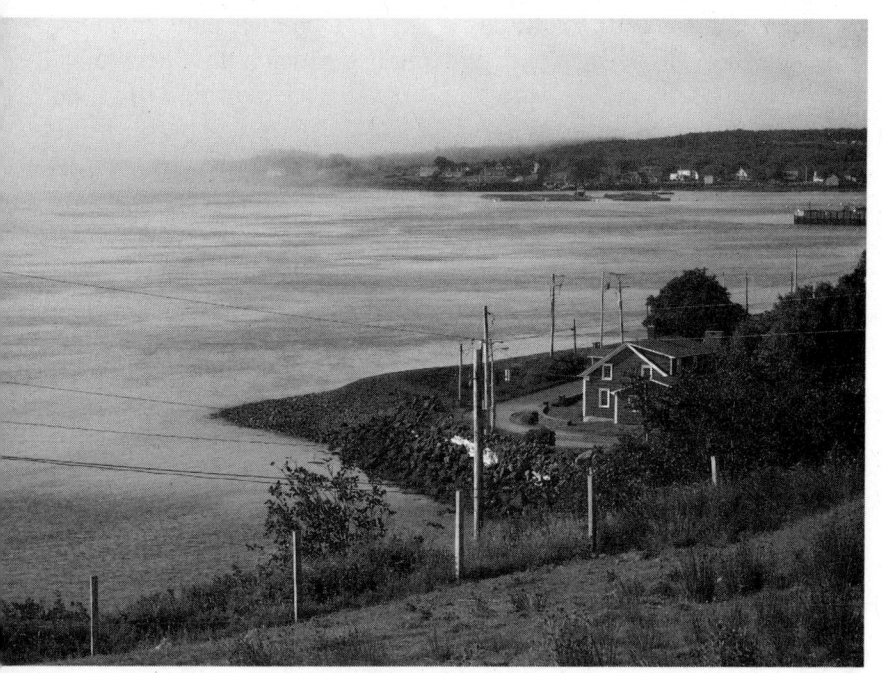

It was a beautiful morning in mid August in 1954. Katie had fed and bathed Ellen, our 2?-month-old daughter, who was now sleeping peacefully in her pink bassinet, close but not too close to the kitchen stove.

Katie and I and Cam, our three-year-old son, were having breakfast. He was a happy, healthy, delightful kid. I often wished out loud that he could stay carefree, content and well fed like that all of his life.

Katie, of course, in addition to her duties as wife and mother, was my receptionist, day planner, emergency standby nurse, assistant, and general factotum. We were talking about prioritizing my house calls for the day when our telephone party line rang. Two short rings was the doctor's house phone. Other people had various combinations of two or three short and/or long rings, but it was a party line and in a perfect world a party-line phone would be answered only in response to one's own specific ring.

However, such was not the practice on the islands. Islanders, curious to hear the news and discover who was sick enough to call the doctor, would impulsively lift the receiver when they heard our two short rings. But, when more than one receiver was picked up, the voice transmission became progressively weaker. When that happened, Elsie – "telephone central" – would order the interlopers to get off the line.

The telephone of the day was a big oak box with a truncated, funnel-shaped device for speaking into and a flashlight-shaped handle listening device that was attached to a cord and hung on a hook on the side of the box.

It was about 8:30 in the morning when Elsie called. Her voice came through clearly at first but as others on the party line clicked in to listen, she barked, "Get off the line, I want to talk to the doctor."

Elsie then told me she had several calls for me. They were not urgent but she wanted to put them through. She knew I had been up until 3 a.m. because of the "exploded vessel" in Central Grove. I didn't need to ask how she knew I had been out that late. There was a well-known island legend that if any man anywhere on the island got up in the middle of the night, walked a mile into the woods and peed behind a tree, in the morning, Hilda Bates, the islands' quintessential gossip and know-it-all, could tell you which tree.

The night before, sometime near midnight, Katie and I were asleep when the phone rang two short blasts. It was surreptitiously and strategically placed on Katie's side of the bed so she answered it. I heard her say, "Explosion! Vessel? What kind of vessel? A ship? In a house? Where?" Then she handed me the phone.

A very agitated male voice screamed that he needed me immediately at a house in Central Grove. I realized later the caller had been making a futile attempt to doubletalk his way past Elsie so she, and anyone else listening in, wouldn't know what had happened.

I grabbed my medical bag and another one with whatever surgical tools I had and rushed off to Central Grove. I found the house and the agitated and terrified young man. He was in his mid 30s, small, wiry and half dressed. His wife, a new bride the day before, in response to nature's call had risen during the wedding night and, not having indoor plumbing, used the pot under the bed.

Now that particular instrument had been variously named "the jug", "the thunder jug", or, in Cape Breton, "the guzzunder", and was usually made of either metal or crockery. In this instance, it was, or rather had been an antique Limoges pot brought from the old country by an early settler to New England some 200 years before, and later by United Empire Loyalists to the Digby Islands. It had performed well hundreds of times previously but now, with age and multiple stress fractures, it had become the central prop in a very personal, emotional and embarrassing melodrama.

The bride was a rather hefty young woman whose weight on the antique Limoges pot caused it to shatter into 1,000 pieces, with resultant multiple lacerations and shards and fragments of glass and porcelain being embedded in places I had never imagined such things should, or could, ever be found.

That was the "explosion of the vessel" in Central Grove.

In the dead of night on this small, windswept, fog-bound

island, transport to hospital was not an option. Handling the situation was the duty of the country doctor, the healer, the hope of those in need, so, leaping into the breach, so to speak, I positioned the dispirited blushing bride face down on her bed over a large bolster with only her bare posterior exposed and pointing to the heavens. She was crying and in pain.

My patient was partly comforted by a quarter grain of morphine – chloroform was an ideal anaesthetic for short procedures but contra indicated in long ones – and this was going to take some time. I reverted to the old country doctor's effective standby... three ounces of Johnnie Walker Scotch. I suspected her sobbing might really have been a crying jag from the booze.

For the next three hours of his wedding night, under the light of a flickering kerosene lamp, a flashlight and several candles, a distraught bridegroom stood by, moving and shifting the various lights to reflect the myriad shards of glass and porcelain for me to pick out of his bride's behind.

During this time, I couldn't help reflecting on my boyhood dreams of the glamour, excitement and thrill of becoming a medical doctor, ministering to the sick and afflicted, being revered in the community, hailed as a champion of those in need. I even recalled the comment of my dreamy eyed, overly romantic mother: "People will want to touch the hem of your garment."

I wasn't long in realizing the life of a country doctor was not all glamour, that there are occasional unpleasant tasks that make you wonder, "Is this really where I want to be?"

Indeed, there are disappointments and failures but there are so many more exhilarating, satisfying, happy and pleasant occasions... like being the first to hold and hear a healthy newborn baby cry, like bringing a child through a pneumonia crisis, or seeing a loved and elderly grandmother recover from a heart attack.

On balance, it was all worthwhile. But have no illusions, the life and responsibilities of the isolated country doctor were very different from those of his boyhood memories of Dr. Kildare, movies, and the academic life in medical school. It was certainly nothing like the multiple television versions.

As I sutured the last laceration I felt it was great to be there, performing a necessary service and, with the unfounded confidence of youth, I assured myself that I was still the best qualified person to do what had to be done.

Elsie's morning messages were more mundane. The calls were from Westport where, there being no secrets and certainly no privacy laws, I was told Mrs. Bower's hemorrhoids needed attention and, at McDormand's Fish Plant a box had fallen on a man's foot and another had a fishhook in his hand, but the big news of the day was the scandal.

"You know that attractive young woman, Nellie Denton?" Elsie asked.

"Sure," I said, "I delivered her baby a year ago."

"Well, she just left her three kids and run off with Isabel Thurber's husband. He has three kids too."

"I know Nellie and her kids, and her husband," I said. "I treated them all for chickenpox a couple of months ago."

So off I went to Westport. The ferryman, Charlie Webber, a pleasant, delightful, elderly grandfather type, knew about the scandal and was disgusted with such behaviour in the young generation.

"I don't like to say anything bad about nobody," he commented, "but that fella just ain't no good."

I never took my car to Westport. The ferry without a car took much less time and there was only a mile and a half of road on the island anyway. Several cars were always around the ferry dock and Raymond Robichaud's general store.

One of the drug companies had supplied me with sample vitamins in 1?-ounce bottles. Having the habits of a cautious, canny and penurious Scot, I transferred these samples in larger bottles and peddled them to patients. I saved the small bottles and filled them with rum or scotch. Whenever I offered one, suddenly a number of cars were at my disposal.

After doing whatever had to be done with Mrs. Bower, McDormand's Fish Plant was next. The fish hook was about three inches long and embedded in the man's left hand, with a piece of line still attached. It could not be backed out because of the barb so, with my trusty heavy duty pliers, especially acquired and sterilized for this oft-repeated situation, I cut the loop off the hook, injected Novocain into the skin at the exit site and, using the pliers as a surgical needle driver, drove the point of the hook through the anaesthetized skin. Then, grabbing the point of the hook with the pliers, I pulled the thing out. There was no real risk of infection.

The fisherman's usual immediate first aid in fish hook injuries was to immerse the wound in a bucket of gasoline but, with all due respect to folklore, I also added a shot of penicillin.

The man with the foot problem had only soft tissue bruising and no fracture. When I told Melbourne McDormand there was no serious injury but that it was the biggest and dirtiest foot I had ever seen, his reply was, "You ain't never seen his father's."

With my calls finished, I went to see Nellie Denton's parents. They were even more shocked and surprised at Nellie's abrupt departure than the rest of us were. During our conversation, I mentioned that I thought I knew Nellie quite well. I had seen her and her children often. She shared many confidences with me as her family doctor and I thought she had a happy home and a good marriage.

Nellie's dad, a big, confident, friendly man, a life-long Bay of Fundy fisherman and homespun philosopher, had just finished folding his trawl. Still wearing his big thigh-high rubber boots folded below the knee, he wanted to talk. He reminisced about Nellie's childhood, growing up, her marriage and his grandchildren all living nearby. Life was good so why did this have to happen?

I, too, wondered what a group of experts – academics, psychologists, psychiatrists, social workers, family law lawyers and other specialists, all sitting around a boardroom table – would make of it. None of them, never having experienced life for prolonged periods on a small island, hemmed in by peer pressure, tides, strict religious teaching, married with three kids, diapers, chickenpox, measles and whooping cough, would or could understand why a beautiful young woman in the prime of her life might ask herself, "Is this all there is?"

Complicating this scenario, modern technology had just made

available that new, seductive thing called television. The picture was black and white and the box had rabbit ears, but it showed the glamorous life, the fun, the romance and excitement in the outside world. The contrast with Brier Island was shocking.

The experts would have analyzed, dissected and done a double-blind study fit for a master's thesis, published a long-winded report that would be filed away in a university library and not be of much use to Nellie Denton at any rate.

Nellie's father, a pragmatic, no nonsense independent thinker not having had the advantage or contamination of higher learning, summed it all up in 10 words: "I dunno but I guess her ass run away wit her brains." That said it all. There was no need for further analysis.

I left her dad with two small bottles of my special whiskey vitamin replacement and returned to the ferry, confident in the knowledge that as long as clear and realistic thinkers like that were still around, the grassroots would be in good hands.

CHAPTER TWELVE

The Economics and Rationale
of Rural Medicine (before Medicare)

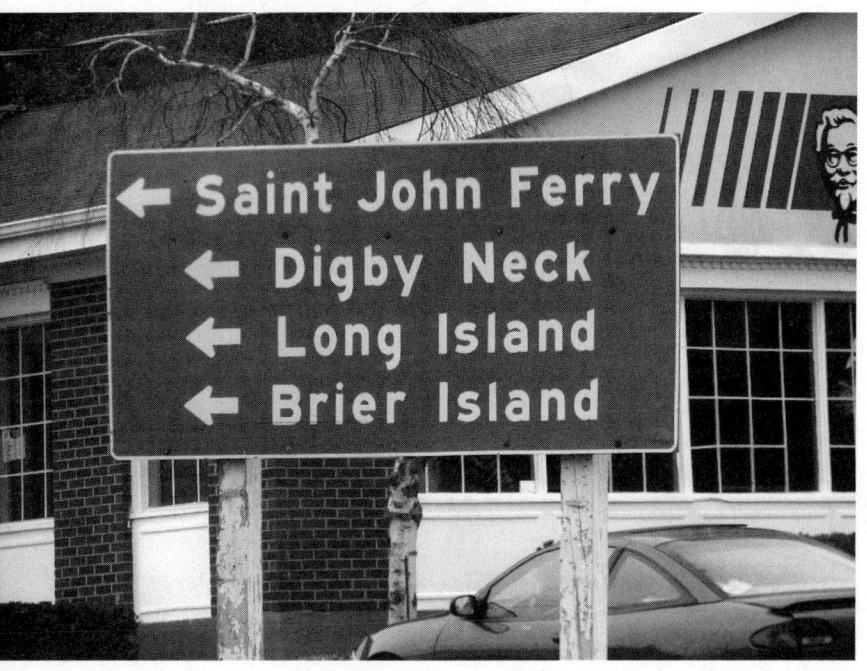

Business training is the best kept secret in medical schools. To medical ethicists, money is a dirty word and should never be a consideration in the provision of medical care.

It used to be taught, and was still a chapter in Yates's Textbook of Medicine when I was a student, that a medical doctor should behave not unlike a monk, that he should never expect money for providing medical service. It was reasonable for the doctor to accept barter in the form of chickens, fish or produce, but only when the patient had recovered... when he would be so grateful he would force money into the hands of his doctor.

With this training, or brain washing, and having been a hospital intern for the past year at $25 a month and living off my pregnant wife's meagre salary as a hospital dietitian, I ventured into the position of country doctor not having the faintest idea how to charge for my services.

Living in a poor fishing village, our lifestyle was not lavish. I had a car, bought for $50 a month, a rented house at $25 a month, and a pregnant wife with no job. Somehow it all had to be financed but I had no idea how to go about it, and no one to ask.

My first call to Tiverton, 10 miles away at the opposite end of the island from Freeport, was to attend to an elderly lady with pneumonia. I had a free sample package of 10 doses of that new drug called penicillin, not only the drug of choice at the time but also the only one available. I made the trip six times, giving a shot of penicillin each time.

The patient's residence was an old, run down wooden house, obviously needing repair and renovation. Her husband was an elderly retired fisherman working as a fish cutter in the local canning factory. As the lady recovered, the husband asked how much he owed me. I surveyed the situation and thought: six visits at 10 miles each, the penicillin was a free sample, the household was decidedly poor, my training in medical ethics weighed heavily, but I also had bills to pay. After some soul searching, I asked for $10.

The husband was surprised my charge was so low. He moved over beside the oil stove in his kitchen, reached for and took down a teapot from the top shelf and produced a $50-bill. In my lifetime, I had never even seen a $50-bill. I couldn't change it... so I never got my $10.

In the outside world, lobster is an expensive luxury. When we arrived in Freeport, we were treated to a lobster dinner. Katie was embarrassed that in a poor fishing village they would serve such expensive fare. We soon learned barter would become a substantial part of my income.

In that area, lobster season was December 1 to May 30. Two or three times a week, I was presented with a sack of 20 or 30 lobsters. I had a garage with a loft where I could spill out the live lobsters to crawl around until we decided to cook them. We had lobster dinners three or four times a week, often alternating with Digby scallops or the freshest fish in the world. We froze or canned the excess. As one old islander told me, "It don't get no better than this."

The only bad feature was that the lobsters were under market size and by law should not have been harvested. Since the practice was illegal, the occasional visit by a Fisheries inspector or an RCMP officer triggered an all-island warning. Elsie would make strategic phone calls so everybody knew, and all became involved in a conspiracy of silence. The practice of selling lobster under market size was certainly detrimental to the lobster industry but it had gone on for decades. Fortunately, it has since been discontinued.

In my first year in practice I saw my first case of poliomyelitis. I had heard there were polio cases in Nova Scotia and a polio clinic had been set up in the Infectious Diseases Hospital in Halifax. The diagnosis of my first patient wasn't difficult: a 14-year-old girl with headache, fever, stiff neck and leg muscle spasm. I bundled the child into my car, called Katie and told her I was off to Halifax.

This was my first of seven cases. I took them all to Halifax in my own car because I felt no one else was qualified in case of emergency, and it was my duty as a doctor. Furthermore, I couldn't justify charging money for transporting a friend and neighbour in an emergency. Fortunately, most of the cases recovered with only minor sequelae... and I got a whole lot more lobster.

One evening just before dark, I received an urgent call to go and see a 12-year-old girl. She was in severe muscle spasm, head, neck and back fully arched and extended, the so called opisthotinous position. I made a snap diagnosis of bulbar poliomyelitis and figured this child would require an iron lung before morning. Knowing the ferry did not transport cars after dark and we had no time to waste, I called to have the ferry wait for me. We had to get off the island!

With the kid and her mother along I raced off to Halifax, arriving at the clinic about midnight. The child seemed a little less spastic. In the morning, I went back to the clinic to see her. She had no more muscle spasm, looked well and was happily eating breakfast. Then the junior intern came to me and, with a snide grin and sarcastic tone, told me I should go back to medical school to learn to recognize the difference between poliomyelitis and an epileptic seizure!

So, more than a little embarrassed, I took the child home. I would like to have bragged that I had facilitated a miraculous cure but thought honesty the better choice. However, if ever faced with the same situation, a sick child, the threat of bulbar polio and no ferry after dark, I'd still make the dash for Halifax.

My next lesson in rural economics came from the operators of the two general stores in Tiverton. One was run by Louie Elliott and his sister Annabelle, both young, energetic, able bodied, enthusiastic and interesting people. In addition to the store, they had an Esso gasoline pump. Every house on the island had an oil burning stove, and Louie had the oil contract.

Annabelle was a stocky, tomboy type with a crooked grin, the result of childhood Bell's Palsy. She was able to handle any situation, from pumping gas to lifting and tossing five-gallon glass containers of stove oil into the back of the pickup truck, cutting meat, selling groceries and fishing gear, demonstrating tools, and custom fitting clothes. In this latter regard, when a customer complained that a hat was too small, Annabelle took it into the back room, put it on her own head and with a hefty pull, enlarged it to a perfect fit.

All the fishing boats in the Tiverton Harbour were painted beige. On one occasion when my mother, who had a flair for the quaint and elegant, came to visit, she commented on how nice it was to have such good community spirit and cooperation. "Such a pretty scene to have those charming little boats all the same colour."

Little did mother know that Louie Elliott was the only supplier of paint in the village and he only brought in one colour, which he called "beege".

The other general store was owned by Elbridge Outhouse, a big elderly man, obese, friendly, and a great storyteller and philosopher. He sat on a high stool behind an old scratched, semi-frosted glass showcase with a worn, chipped and battered wooden frame containing chocolate bars and penny candy.

The two stores were in friendly competition and each had its own coterie of customers. I visited both and one day, while talking to Elbridge, a customer came in and complained that Elbridge was selling canned Heinz Pork and Beans for 17 cents a can, but Louie Elliott, 300 yards away, was charging only 16 cents.

Elbridge leaned over the old glass showcase and quietly made the classic statement: "Louie ain't makin' so much money as me."

Dr. Andrew Weir, who had practised medicine on the islands, became my mentor in both medicine and financial management. He provided me with a simple fee schedule and advised that invoices for medical services were never mailed in the country the way they were in city practices. "Here," he said, "you make out your bills and carry them with you to present the next time you make a call, or when you just happen to be passing by."

On one occasion, he said he had to be quite gruff with a patient who said he couldn't pay the bill because Christmas was coming.

"Christmas is coming for me too," Dr. Weir replied.

I was never that brave.

When Dr. Weir was planning to retire, his son Eddie had just graduated from Dalhousie Medical School and came to relieve his father on the islands for one year.

During that time, when Dr. Weir came back to visit, the son chided his father, facetiously reporting that after the father had treated old Mrs. Mattie Teed for years for asthma, he, the son, had finally cured her.

The old doc calmly replied, "You shouldn't have done that son; her asthma put you through college."

It was reported to me that the young Dr. Weir was really smart because he used big words all the time, and therefore "must be a really good doctor." Knowing that information is power, and with that as my clue, the next call I had was to a big strapping, able-bodied fisherman, so big he could be afraid of nothing in this world. He looked like he could wrestle alligators.

He had a bad cold, aches and pains and a low grade fever. After examining him, I gave him the usual aspirin, cough medicine and a horrible gargle mixture made with dobel tablets dissolved in water. When he asked what my diagnosis was, I seized on the lesson from young Dr. Weir and said, "You've got upper respiratory infection, with pyrexia, malaise and polymyositis."

That big, burly strong man went pale, almost into shock.

"Geez" he asked, "is that anything like the flu?"

I realized the big words almost scared him to death and replied, "Yes, it's just like the flu." All of which goes to prove an old island proverb: "Sometimes book learnin' just ain't that helpful."

The senior Dr. Weir gave me another clue to success as a country doctor.

"Never," he said, "under any circumstance, try to treat animals. If you treat a dog and it doesn't recover, they will never let you treat their kids." So, he suggested, "let your wife be the veterinarian."

Taking this advice to heart, I obtained a small pamphlet on veterinary medicine from a drug company and appointed Katie to be in charge of veterinary services.

Time passed, but eventually Katie's big test came.

Mr. Pugh, the local dairy farmer, called Katie for help. He had a sick cow with a severe udder infection. Katie rose to the challenge.

"Do you have any sulfa drug? she asked.

"Yes," was his reply. He had a drum of it in the barn but the label with the dosage on it was worn off.

Katie asked how much the cow weighed.

"About 800 to 900 pounds," Mr. Pugh replied.

Katie is a professional dietitian, expert at calculating calories, carbohydrates, proteins and fats in grams per hundredweight for humans, but beyond that, mathematics was just not her strong suit.

The veterinary pamphlet gave a chart of dosages for animals calculated in "stones". A "stone" is an old English weight measure ranging anywhere from five to 14 pounds, but in old veterinary circles it was generally accepted as equal to about 13.5 pounds. With all her education, Katie had never heard of "stone" as a measurement of weight. In reading the pamphlet, she assumed a stone was just a veterinary term for pound and ordered Mr. Pugh to give the cow half an ounce of sulfa per pound for 900 pounds.

Mr. Pugh argued that that sounded like a big dose but Katie's veterinary expertise was not to be challenged.

"That's a severe infection in a big animal, and it has to be treated aggressively," she said.

Mr. Pugh blinked but followed instructions. The cow developed a bowel obstruction caused by an overdose of sulfa and died two days later.

Mr. Pugh called and Katie responded with unjustified and unshaken confidence: "Sorry to hear that, next time you better call me earlier," she said.

He never did.

CHAPTER THIRTEEN
Family Influences

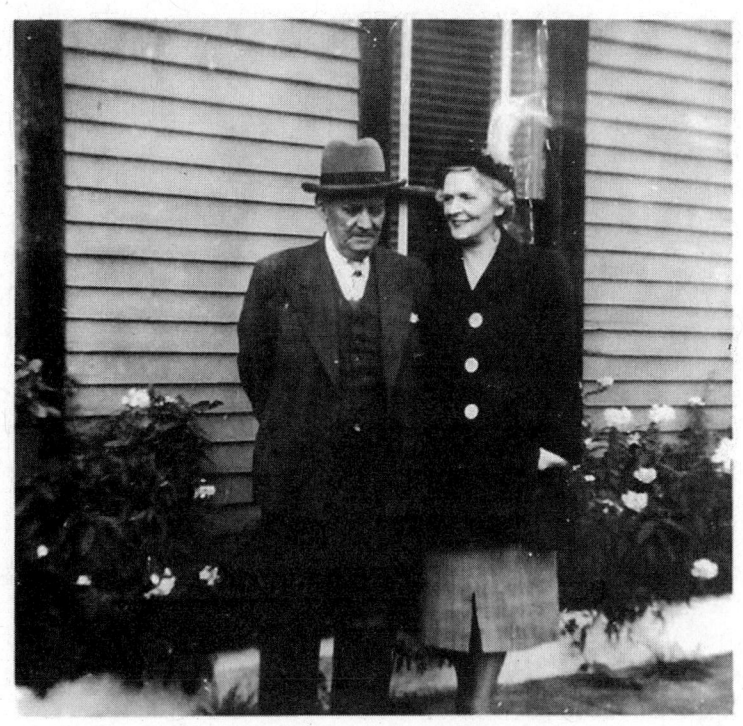

While Katie and I felt confident and independent in our new life, we were still young and immature, and whether we knew it or not, we did have an emotional need for a measure of family backup.

My father had died three years before we went to the Islands. Mother lived in Halifax. She was a retired teacher and actor and was still working as a radio broadcaster. Mother was charming, engaging, loveable, egocentric, and impossible to live with. She had to be centre stage, managing and manipulating everyone in her presence. Katie and I thought we should be in command.

Katie had been one of mother's not-so-favoured students at university. It would be charitable to say they did not like each other, a situation that was compounded by the fact that at our wedding, Kate's mother and my mother appeared in identical dresses and each insisted the other go back to the hotel and change.

My mother visited us on the Islands frequently, came with me to sit in the car while I made house calls, and charmed every islander she met. Mother, often critical of her daughter-in-law's management of home and children, had difficulty understanding that this was Katie's home and she was a guest in it. But despite the built-in conflicts, our kids loved their grandmother and now, having grown up, Katie and I can laugh at the old problems and, in retrospect, can even find enjoyment in recollecting those visits.

Katie's mother came to visit only once to oversee the decoration and furnishing of our house but found the shopping opportunities in our three general stores not like those in the big cities. After all, how much interest could an elegant lady have in hay, oats fishnets and marine hardware?

We had much more friendly and enjoyable contact with Katie's father, who was one of the most interesting, fascinating and delightful personalities I have ever met. He came across the Bay of Fundy from Saint John frequently and provided the family support we didn't know we needed. The following is a short biography of this wonderful man.

Captain William Traynor was a master mariner, a ship's captain, and when I met him, he had been a pilot in Saint John

Harbour and the Bay of Fundy for more than 30 years. William Traynor grew up on the Bay of Fundy, went to sea as a boy, became a ship's master, captain, and eventually a pilot in the Bay of Fundy, which he loved and knew very well.

As a boy, he and his father would row a dory out into the bay to meet an incoming ship. The dory would be hoisted onto the deck of the ship and the old man, knowing the tides, currents, effect of the wind force and direction, shoals and other hazards, would then pilot the ship into harbour at Saint John, New Brunswick.

In winter, when the air is much colder than the water, dense fog rises more than 50 feet above the sea. The man and boy in the dory had no means of contacting their incoming ship and if they missed it, they had no choice but to continue to row the rest of the 50 miles to the shore of Nova Scotia. Their only provisions were pipe tobacco, a flat of salt codfish, and a keg of rum. Running out of salt cod or rum was not a problem but being out of tobacco was a serious matter.

Over the years, the pilot service became more organized and equipped with government-supplied boats resembling tugboats. They performed well with the expert seamanship and know-how that came only with experience and study of the rapidly changing and often violent moods of the bay. The pilots worked in teams of two, one would operate the pilot boat to meet an incoming ship, the other would grab onto and climb a rope ladder to the ship's deck, then proceed to the bridge to pilot the ship into harbour.

The pilots, naturally, became the search and rescue service on the Bay of Fundy. During the Second World War, young, partially trained lieutenants of the Canadian navy, with their new commissions, bravado and unfounded confidence, learned to sail in the relatively predictable waters off the coast of Halifax and would rent small sailboats to go into the Bay of Fundy.

They had been taught to sail up wind on the first leg of a pleasure sail in order to make for an easier and safer return. But the Bay of Fundy tides, freaky winds, currents and waves change all that. When the young sailors were reported overdue and missing, the call invariably came into the pilot office. Will Traynor, or his veteran pilot partner Fen McKelvey, would ask from where and when they had left. Then, knowing the tide direction, currents and wind direction, they would know exactly where to pick up the frightened, humbled sailors – and their even more terrified girl-friends.

When I met Captain Will Traynor he was in his early 60s, short in stature, dedicated; he had a dominant personality and was one of the best storytellers I have ever met. He had the heartiest laugh ever heard and loved to recount tales of shipwrecks in the Bay of Fundy, and there were lots of them. He once said that during the Great Depression (There was nothing great about it), children going to bed would pray, being good Irish Catholic kids: "God bless Momma and Poppa and send a ship ashore tonight."

He told stories of fishermen scavengers stripping a grounded freighter, filling their dories and boats with food, furniture and ship's fixtures. On one occasion, a piano was lowered onto a dory then played by an inebriated fisherman while his buddy sang and rowed the boat. This lasted until they came upon a floating cask of Demerara rum. When they reached for the rum, overboard went the piano and inboard came the rum.

I was a young medical doctor, married to Will Traynor's daughter and about to go into practice. I marveled at his ability to do his job. He stood barely five feet tall and was stocky, hyperten-sive, diabetic and had coronary artery disease and thyrotoxicosis. He had had two previous heart attacks. Yet, with all that, he was able to grab onto and climb a 50-foot rope ladder swinging from the side of a moving freighter while wearing a three-piece suit, shirt and tie, a full overcoat and homburg hat.

Will would get to the deck of the freighter and have to lie down long enough to get his breath before making the next climb to the wheelhouse. Once there, taking command of the ship, he'd give the order, "Half speed ahead and lay off two points to star-board (or larboard)", all the while puffing on his ever-present pipe full of Old Chum tobacco.

He was a pleasant and easy-to-talk-to man, a second-genera-tion descendant of the Irish culture of County Cork in Southern Ireland. He was also colourful and eloquent, witty and funny, with an unlimited fund of stories, expressions and salty language from years at sea in barques, brigantines, steam and diesel-driven sailing ships.

Will Traynor was married to Kathleen Daly, a beautiful, elegant lady with an unequalled sense of propriety. She was nicknamed "Kit" by Will. Will also had a sister, Francie, a dominant, stocky Victorian woman who taught Grade 2 in the Catholic School system and could have easily qualified as an unforgiving mother superior.

Will's father had been a Saint John Harbour pilot for 40 years, had an unblemished record of bringing ships in and out of the harbour, and a reputation for drinking hard liquor. That feature weighed heavily on Kit and Francie, who decreed that drinking of alcohol would never be permitted in their generation. Together, they forbade any type of booze in their households.

Meanwhile, it was the custom for the captain of a ship coming from a foreign port to present the local pilot with a bottle of liquor from his home country. The bottle was often a fancy decanter with a flamboyant label and a colourful ribbon. Will would bring this bottle home and watch patiently while Kit opened it and poured the contents down the kitchen sink. She would then place the decorative bottle on a high shelf in the kitchen with all the others.

I knew Will loved a drink of gin and whenever he came to Freeport I'd have an adequate supply to share... just one of the reasons he came often. I marveled at his tolerance of the disposal of all that high quality foreign booze until one Christmas evening after he had just been discharged from hospital after his second heart attack.

There was an unopened bottle of high quality Irish whiskey under the Christmas tree. Kit had told me earlier that she had, in sympathy for Will's condition, left that bottle unmolested, thinking it might make him feel better just knowing it was there but, since he had not even mentioned it, maybe he was "just not recovering from the heart attack." She denied my suggestion that she might be mellowing after all those years of addiction to temperance.

In the quiet of the evening, I whispered to Will that he and I should get into that elegant bottle of Irish whiskey. Will looked around to be sure no one was listening and whispered back: "Cam, it's not whiskey any more... it's tea."

It was then I realized that all that beautiful booze that had been poured down the Traynor kitchen sink over many years had already been consumed by the pilots and replaced with some colourful, harmless liquid. The elegant cut glass decanters were still being proudly displayed on the high kitchen shelf.

Will visited Freeport often. He was comfortable in our house. After all, his wife, the quintessential homemaker, had furnished and decorated it. She had used her daughter's new home as an excuse to get all new stuff for her own house and ship the older but still beautiful furniture to Freeport. Katie and I were most grateful.

Will, looking around our living room, recognized all his own furniture, drapes, carpets and even knickknacks. The difference was that at our house he could have a drink of gin. He was a most welcome guest and we looked forward to his coming every time.

Will would cross the Bay of Fundy on a small costal freight boat called the Tagati, which looked like the boat in the movie African Queen. It was owned and operated solely by Angus Dakin. Both boat and operator were rather unkempt. Dakin was a wiry little man, tough as nails, and sailed alone, making weekly trips around the periphery of the Bay of Fundy delivering freight to small costal ports. Will was the only passenger he ever took.

Angus Dakin was also a severe epileptic and when out in the bay, if he felt the prodromes of a seizure coming on, he'd head the boat toward open water, lash down the helm and lie down in his bunk with a piece of wood between his teeth, and wait. When the seizure was over, he'd figure out from his compass direction, from the tide and speed of the boat just where he was and resume his deliveries.

On one occasion on board the Tagati, Dakin and Will were motoring south on the ebb tide. They saw a storm coming out of the Atlantic from the southeast. Knowing the wind blowing in opposite direction to the tide stirs up stormy seas, they battened down, kept their course for Brier Island light and made ready for rough water. As the storm hit and the little boat was thrown about,

Dakin felt the prodromes of an epileptic seizure, thrust his trusty piece of wood between his teeth and threw himself onto his bunk.

Will grabbed the helm, but even with all his sea-going experience he had never seen a full blown grand mal convulsion. He thought he had to do something and momentarily left the helm to look at Dakin. The boat broached in the wild sea. Will grabbed the helm again, got the boat under control and thought for sure Dakin, still convulsing, was going to die and it would be all his fault because he had done nothing to help. But Dakin didn't die. He recovered as he always had, took control of his boat and arrived as scheduled in Freeport.

I met the Tagati at Fish Point wharf. Will was still quite shaken. I had to remind him that Dakin had done this many times before and, scary as it was, he had had everything under control. There was nothing Will could have done to help. The take-home message here was that when anyone says he has seen it all and that there are no more surprises in life, you can be sure he has never been to sea or practised medicine in the country.

We have many happy memories of Will Traynor, his good nature, his stories, his hearty laugh and generosity. We loved him dearly and were crushed on the morning of January 14, 1957, when his life came to a tragic end. The following is a speculative, fictionalized account of what might have happened that fateful day.

At 2 a.m., January 14, 1957, Will Traynor's alarm clock woke him to greet a new day. Pilot Boat No. 1, with three other pilots, an apprentice pilot, an engineer, a cook and a deckhand on board, was scheduled to leave the dock at Reed's Point at 5 a.m. They were to cross Saint John Harbour, drop off a pilot to take a ship out on the ebbing tide, then proceed to station a mile west of Fairway Buoy in the Bay of Fundy, close to the approach to Saint John Harbour.

Will Traynor, showered, shaved and fully dressed in his usual three-piece suit, shirt, tie, overcoat and homburg, looked at the outside temperature, tapped the barometer, and ventured out. Reed's Point was a mile and a half away. The temperature was 23 degrees Fahrenheit below freezing. Will thought of trying to start his old Oldsmobile but the air was so cold and the fog so thick he couldn't even see the radiator ornament from the driver's seat. It was safer to walk in extremely cold weather... even for a 68-year-old man with severe coronary artery disease, hypertension and thyrotoxicosis. He wrapped his scarf around his face and set out on foot. He was tough and dedicated and made the trip red faced and breathless, but he got there.

With the air temperature that cold and the Bay of Fundy water just above 32 degrees, dense fog rose 50-100 feet above sea level. The pilot boat was an 80-foot, low-freeboard wooden vessel with a powerful engine and experienced crew. Ideally suited for its role of getting a pilot aboard an incoming ship, the pilot boat would be manoeuvred around to the leeside of the ship where the pilot would grab a rope ladder and climb 50 feet up to the deck, then to the bridge.

To take a pilot off an outbound ship, the pilot would climb down the rope ladder to the heaving deck of the pilot boat. When the weather was too rough to get off, the pilot was carried to the ship's next port.

The wheelhouse of Pilot Boat No. 1 was 15-17 feet above the waterline. Visibility was severely limited by the ice fog but these men didn't rely only on visibility. They also navigated by tide, current and wind. These pilots were cautious but undaunted. For them, this was just another day of travelling in fog. The Bay of Fundy, they boasted, made fog like this and shipped it all over the world.

With no difficulty, the pilot was dropped off on the west side of the harbour and Pilot Boat No. 1 proceeded to its position at Fairway Buoy to await the arrival of the ship, the Fort Avalon, expected within the next two hours. While waiting, the sweet smell of bacon and eggs, strong coffee and Old Chum pipe tobacco filled the boat, along with camaraderie and embellished sea yarns. They told of experiences sailing around the world, captains they had known, shipwrecks, disasters, near disasters and funny stories, all the while keeping a sharp lookout, unable to see anything but listening over the howling wind for any sound of a ship. They could hear and see nothing.

The Fort Avalon was inbound to Saint John Harbour. She had been there before and, with unfounded confidence, the skipper was nonchalant. Despite the dense fog, he proceeded at 14 knots. His radar showed a small blip... The helmsman paid no attention. According to their dead reckoning, they were approaching Fairway Buoy.

In fact, they were off course a mile and a quarter to the west, on a direct collision course with Pilot Boat No. 1. When the 50-foot-high bow of the Fort Avalon was 10 feet away from the starboard side of the pilot boat, the pilot at the helm called for "full astern," but it was too late. The steel bow of the big ship crashed through the port side of the pilot boat just forward of the wheelhouse. The heavy oak timbers of the small boat were splintered like matchsticks, no match for the big heavy freighter still travelling at 14 knots.

The noise was deafening. The sound of the collision combined with the shattering of glass in the wheelhouse, the scattering of everything not tied down, the tossing of the crew to the starboard side, the men's cries: "Christ, we've been hit! Gawddamn it! We're goin' over," and Will Traynor's booming voice bellowing, "All hands make for the port side door!"

As the cabin filled with icy water, the bow of the Avalon crushed to the keelson of the pilot boat and rolled her over, turned her turtle and ran her under the keel, sending the pilot boat to the bottom of the Bay of Fundy with all seven lives. The Bay of Fundy, once cherished, loved, respected and feared by seven expert seamen, now claimed them all forever.

Fifty years to the day after the worst tragedy in the long history of the Saint John Pilot Service, January 14, 2007, a memorial ceremony was held to commemorate the lives of the seven men who drowned at the junction of the Bay of Fundy and Saint John Harbour.

Realizing we all must die sometime, Will Traynor, while he pretended to hate farmers and undertakers, had attended every Irish wake in Saint John and county, helping to stand the corpse in the corner with a drink in its hand while mourners danced and drank to his health and new life in the hereafter. Will died in the

Bay of Fundy that he loved so well, and thus avoided the undertaker he never liked. I can imagine him now, sitting at a seaside bar in heaven, his foot on the brass rail with a glass of gin and a pipe full of Old Chum tobacco, telling stories to Saint Peter, who was also a sailor, laughing and ordering a big dish of strawberry shortcake.

The service was organized by the chief pilot Don Duffy and lawyer Neil McKelvey, son of a retired pilot. These two men then decided to research and write the history of the Saint John Pilot Service. The book has now been published.

McKelvey and Duffy needed a name for their book, something that would capture the attention of readers and reflect what a marine pilot does. The pilots, all master mariners, recalled piloting experiences with big and small commercial ships as well as with big naval vessels during the Second World War, in all weather conditions, fog, 30-foot tides, currents and old shipwrecks. The one memory that stood out in everyone's mind was the visit of the QE2 to Saint John.

As the big ship sailed slowly through the Bay of Fundy, the fog got thicker. The bow of the ship could not be seen from the bridge. The Bay of Fundy is the only place in the world where wind does not blow fog away, it just compacts it into confusing shadows, comparable to being lost in a desert and seeing an oasis.

The QE2, the biggest ship in the world, approached Saint John Harbour. The captain, with the sole responsibility for the safety of his ship and some 3,000 passengers and crew on board, now in unfamiliar and dangerous waters, running with a 30-foot tide, zero visibility, and knowing the history of multiple previous shipwrecks, was anxious to meet the local pilot. Never having met him, he wondered about his competence and was uneasy about giving command of his vessel to a complete stranger in a risky situation.

The captain, seasoned, experienced, confident, dominant and in control of Cunard's flagship, the greatest and most beautiful ship, was, to say the least, apprehensive. He had radar, sonar and every type of navigating device known. GPS had not yet been invented. The marine charts often state, "Local knowledge needed here." That was the only thing the QE2 did not have.

The pilot, Don Duffy, also a captain, a master mariner, confident and dominant as the seasoned senior Saint John Harbour pilot, had taken hundreds of ships in and out of this harbour, most of them in fog like the QE2 was facing. But he had never had a prize like the QE2. He did not know how the ship would react, but he did know the harbour.

"Is it safe in this fog?" the ship's captain asked.

"This is Saint John," the pilot replied. "If we didn't work in fog, we wouldn't work at all."

Consider the psychological profiles of the captain and the pilot, standing face to face on the darkened bridge of a multi-million dollar ocean liner with 3,000 people on board, in dense fog, in dangerous water, and committed to a tight schedule of arrival and departure.

The two captains, both competent, experienced titans of the sea, studied each other carefully then stared into the dense fog, both fully aware of their respective responsibilities: one very concerned and apprehensive, the other very confident and assured. A decision had to be made. The captain of the greatest ship in the world finally declared: "She's all yours, Mr. Pilot."

The pilot turned to the helmsman and ordered: "Quarter speed ahead, lay off two points to starboard."

The book of the history of the Saint John Pilot Service was named *She's All Yours Mr. Pilot,* published by Trinity Enterprise Inc., 94 Prince William St., Saint John, NB.

CHAPTER FOURTEEN
Epilogue

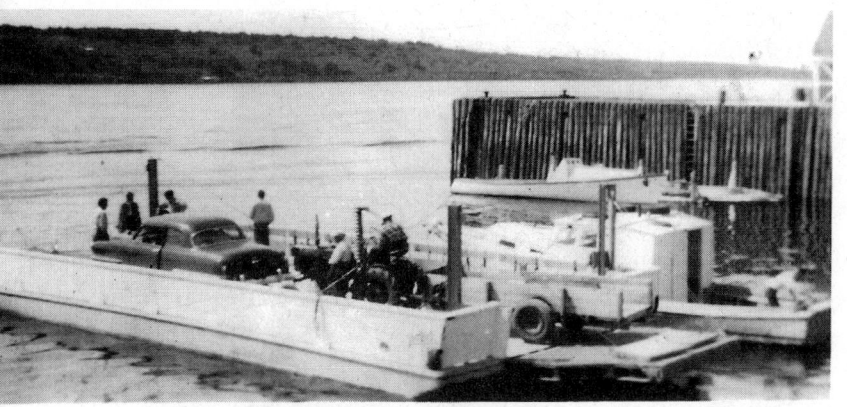

FREEPORT FERRY, FREEPORT, N. S.

My years as a country doctor were some of the happiest and most satisfying of my medical career. The joy of country practice comes from the relationships a doctor develops with his patients, who are also his friends, neighbours and fellow citizens. This is not to belittle the urban doctor whose practice consists predominantly of office visits and hospital duties.

The country doctor's practice consists mainly of house calls, having meals with the family, occasionally staying overnight to sit with a sick child or sleeping on a sofa waiting for a home delivery. The opportunity in country practice to get to know patients, their cares, troubles, likes, dislikes, allergies and idiosyncrasies is unparalleled.

My medical office consisted of two rooms off the kitchen at the back of my house, a small waiting room with four wooden chairs and a slightly larger consulting/examining room big enough for an old wooden examining table and an older desk. Later on, I inherited a retired, small autoclave from the Digby Hospital. It had an electrical short circuit so when I poured the necessary half cup of water into it I got a shock. This went on for two years until Willie, an intellectually disabled young man, came in as a patient, saw me jump with an electrical jolt and showed me that a wire attached to the autoclave and a water pipe would prevent the shock, thereby proving that although this young man might not have been bright, he was not stupid. He was a damn site smarter than I was.

With office staff available to take medical history, blood pressure, temperature and weight, a doctor in an urban medical practice can see as many as 30-50 patients on a busy day. Doing predominantly house calls and, in my case, having the ferry service between islands to contend with, I could see 12-15 in my country practice. I did manage to see 20 patients on one day. Time means nothing in the country. The pace is slow and every day is different.

The country doctor is more than the local medicine man. He becomes the father confessor, minister and advisor on everything from family law and other legal matters to breast feeding and teenage conflicts. And in my practice, it made no difference that I was Roman Catholic and most patients called themselves "hard-shell Baptists".

I learned there was a tremendous difference between the academic and the real world... that compromises are necessary and crises focus your attention. As some great philosopher explained, "Life begins, life goes on, and life ends." The country doctor with limited resources can help but cannot work miracles. His successes are exhilarating, like the seven-year-old child with lobar pneumonia to whom I gave the newly available drug penicillin. He had a fever of 105 degrees and had reached what the old country doctors used to call "the 14-day crisis" – the time when the fever reached a record high point and suddenly began to drop. The patient would either live or die.

I had read about the crisis of lobar pneumonia but had never seen it. From midnight to 4 a.m., I watched helplessly while his temperature fell abruptly from 105 to 93 degrees. The child was cold and shivering. I thought I had lost him. Suddenly, he began to warm up, colour and breathing improved, he was alive and he lived! The family thought I was a hero but I knew that God wanted that kid to survive and perhaps, thereby, also looked after the lonely and scared young country doctor.

Defeats can be crushing, particularly sudden deaths and avoidable accidents, like the death of a young mother from a carelessly stored, loaded shotgun found by a five-year-old child. In subsequent house calls, I made a point of looking for the ever-present shotgun. I found at least seven, each leaning against the wall behind a kitchen stove, all loaded, safety catches off. But it was difficult to counter the argument: "Them old things ain't been fired for years." I would persuade the owner to take the old gun out into the yard, put the butt on the ground, pull the trigger and blast off a shell from the gun he knew was not loaded.

Patients invariably recover from minor illnesses and if that recovery coincides with something the doctor has done, he gets the credit. As one islander verbalized it, "A visit from the doctor is better than a bowl a medicine."

For the country doctor, there are more successes than failures.

The home delivery of a healthy newborn baby is most fulfilling and compensates for any disappointments – worth far more than the $20 he may, or may not be paid for it.

In the 50s, the new concept of "early ambulation" after delivery of a baby was introduced. Prior to that, accepted practice was for the new mother to be confined to bed in a darkened room for two to three weeks. There were two reasons for that custom. The first: "She needed time to get her strength back." The second was rooted in an old religious teaching that "a woman had to be cleansed after child birth." This is still advocated today in some church prayer books.

In my post-natal visits, I often found it necessary to raise blinds, open windows, and even tear off curtains while bellowing like a bombastic preacher that, "God has presented you with a beautiful baby so get out of bed and into the sunshine; enjoy the greatest gift any human being could ever have... and be proud... show your baby to everyone in the world. People will envy you."

The country doctor has opportunities denied his urban colleagues. On one occasion, a friend who was interning at Queen Elizabeth Hospital in Montreal came to visit. At dinner that evening a teenaged boy was brought to my office. He had fallen and had what an orthopaedic surgeon calls a "dinner-fork deformity" of the right wrist, a typical colles fracture. I was able to show my friend a snatch of country medicine.

I had a portable dental X-ray machine that had been converted to take X-rays of small parts. I took a picture, developed it in my back porch, confirmed the diagnosis, gave the lad four drops of chloroform. on a mask, set the fracture and applied a plaster cast. My intern friend, being impressed, commented, "In my hospital in Montreal, I wouldn't be allowed to do that until my second or third year residency."

Later that evening, a call came from Westport. An elderly man with heart trouble was having difficulty breathing, and would I come immediately. Elsie called the ferry for me. My doctor friend and I both went for what I figured might be another demonstration of rural medicine. We boarded the ferry, left the dock on a pleasant night with light fog and a cool breeze.

The ferryman, nicknamed Friday, was tough, not a friendly, happy man, especially since he had just bought "one of them new black and white television sets with rabbit ears and was missing the first hockey game he had ever seen." About half way across Grand Passage, the boat's rudder jammed at about a 30-degree angle, turning the boat to the left in lazy circles while the flood tide swept us north toward the Bay of Fundy. Friday kept trying to straighten the rudder but was unsuccessful. The boat kept getting closer to the rocky cliffs, drifting toward the north-end lighthouse.

As the ragged, rocky wall approached, I began to panic and wondered if it would be possible to climb or even survive on it; we were about to find out. Friday ordered me to go up to the foredeck of the ferry boat to "see if they was an anchor." I found it.

He hollered, "Is they a rope on it?"

I bellowed back, "No, gawddamn it, they ain't," and wanted to hit him with it. When I got back in the cabin, my friend was also in a panic.

As the tidal flow from the Atlantic Ocean passes through the relatively narrow Grand Passage, the speed of the current increases and, as it meets the Bay of Fundy, conflicting currents generate very rough seas through which navigation demands skillful seamanship and a properly functioning boat. We were drifting helplessly in a derelict toward those seas when Friday calmly announced, "When we get there, we'll turn over."

With the sense of impending doom, thinking this must be a dream and could not possibly be happening to me, I remembered I had six 1.5-ounce bottles of Scotch Whiskey in my medical kit, usually saved for emergencies. This would certainly qualify! The three of us downed my whiskey supply as the boat tossed in the rough sea. To paraphrase the proverb, "There are no atheists in foxholes," there are no atheists in impending shipwrecks. We began to pray.

I have come to realize there is a Supreme Being, a power who looks after country people and blesses their doctors. Most people call Him "God". Some even think He is a woman. In this instance, the ubiquitous and ever-present Elsie was His, or Her, agent.

When I did not arrive as promised, the patient's wife called Elsie. Elsie checked with Katie. I had gone. Elsie called Bernie Blackford, who lived near the ferry wharf. He saw my car parked there... and then he saw the light of the ferry boat tossing in the rough water at the north end of the passage close to the lighthouse.

Elsie sent an emergency blast of telephone rings to every telephone in Westport and barked, "The ferry's in trouble at the north end of Grand Passage... and the doctor's on board! Do something!" The village sprang to life.

In a fishing village, when a boat is in trouble, every able-bodied man rushes to his boat to help. In the harbour, the first two got their motors started, each with six able-bodied Bay-of-Fundy-experienced sailors aboard, and charged out to the rescue. It seemed like we were thrown about in the wild and disorganized waves for hours, hanging on for dear life and expecting the worst at any moment.

Then the boat hit something. I thought it was the rock wall and this was the end. A man hollered, "Take a line to the bow."

Two other boats came alongside of us, all of us tossing wildly in the tidal rip of the angry Bay of Fundy. Friday secured the line to the bow cleat of the ferry boat but its rudder was still jammed and pulling to the left, making towing against the current impossible. The second boat came to our starboard side, tossed me a line to fasten to the stern cleat to keep the boat straight. We were saved and began to breathe easier.

The rescuers towed us to the Westport dock where we arrived well after midnight. The dock was crowded. Every man, woman and child on Brier Island turned out to greet us and cheer the men who had risked their lives to save us.

Fortunately, crises like that don't happen often, but when they do, everyone in the village gets involved. The reception was great, and comforting. My doctor friend and I began to regain our composure, thanked everyone and praised our rescuers... and wanted to go home.

Friday boasted that he had never really been scared but his previously ruddy complexion was now even paler than mine.

Some good soul then reminded me that the old man we had set out to visit was "real sick", still needed me, and offered to drive me to the house.

Mr. Hicks was well into his 80s and was having difficulty breathing. He was gurgling, frothing at the mouth, and his legs and belly were swollen with ascites. My doctor friend and I agreed on the diagnosis of congestive heart failure with pulmonary edema. I gave him a diuretic by intramuscular injection and started him on digitalis to slow his heart rate and improve cardiac output. Mrs. Hicks then announced she would prepare a kerosene-and-lard poultice to cover his chest and leave it on overnight. She said she had used it once before and it had cured him.

My medical friend and I looked at this poor man with marginal respiration, gasping for breath, bubbling with water soaked lungs and thought of the horror of subjecting him to the inhalation of kerosene fumes all night long.

"No!" I said. "Do not do that."

She insisted she had done it before and it had cured him. We argued and I finally realized that despite the objection of two qualified physicians, this old girl was going to apply the kerosene and lard poultice as soon as we got out the door. A compromise was necessary. I explained that there would certainly be a conflict between the kerosene and these special new medicines I had just given him.

"He's a very sick man and we don't dare to take any chances... so just give him a small kerosene and lard poultice, no bigger than a postcard, but it will be disastrous to leave it on more than 15 minutes."

She reluctantly agreed. The next morning we went to see Mr. Hicks and found him much improved. Realizing medicine is not an exact science, it is reasonable to ask just what had brought about his recovery. We, professionally trained and qualified physicians, knew beyond a shadow of a doubt that the diuretic and the digitalis had done what we had expected. On the contrary, Mrs. Hicks knew beyond a shadow of a doubt that without the kerosene and lard poultice the old boy would not have lasted the night. Popular opinion in the village was equally divided.

Now, in my twilight time, after 57 years in the practice of medicine, first as a country doctor and later specializing in radiology, it is interesting to reflect on the differences. Both are subject to the regulations of the provincial licensing authority. The country doctor has a slower pace and the opportunity to know, not only his patients' illnesses, but also their trials, tribulations, ambitions and dreams. He is friend, companion, neighbour, and partner in village-hall card games.

To be a successful country doctor one has to like people and want to know them better. He/she has to make independent decisions and often consult with colleagues on difficult cases by telephone. Country medicine is a learning experience; it focuses a doctor's attention and makes him or her live closely with successes, failures, and even mistakes. It requires a certain personality, a willingness to live a simple and rewarding lifestyle as a revered, respected and admired pillar of the community.

In 1950 there was, by today's standards, a relatively confined body of medical knowledge. Today, with modern technology and the explosion of scientific knowledge, specialization is necessary and many specialties are subdivided to the point of doctors knowing more and more about less and less. In this rush for knowledge, information and power, the "whole patient" can be forgotten in comments like, "Doctor, there's a breast biopsy in Room 3," or "there's a colonoscopy in 4."

We are inclined to forget that the patient is a person, lying semi-nude on an examining table, exposed to the gaze of a lot of blasé people she doesn't know. She is alone in a crowd and feels she hasn't a friend in the world. She has been stripped of her clothes, her dignity and personal security. She has been given a wrinkled hospital gown with knotted or missing ties and is, to say the least, worried that the medical tests will reveal something serious… and then who will look after her kids, her husband, their mortgage, and a myriad of other things. No one seems to care – unless there's a family doctor involved.

The country doctor would already know the family situation, their worries, their aspirations, and even the family dog! His is the shoulder to lean on. He is the consultant, the interpreter of the test results, the friend in need; he fills the adopted and trusted grandfather role. He is not only needed, he is wanted and more depended upon than anyone else in the whole world... and that makes country medicine very rewarding.

The specialist in medicine provides the expert knowledge required in today's complex medical world. Patients are referred to him/her by other doctors and he/she reports back to a family doctor, who then reports to the person most concerned, the apprehensive patient. This reporting practice, in my view, having been both a country general practitioner in an isolated community and a specialist in a moderately sized city, is more satisfying as a country doctor.

At the risk of causing controversy, it is my considered opinion that all medical graduates, whatever field they choose, should spend some part of their internship or residency as a country doctor in order to develop sensitivity to the needs and souls of the people they will treat for the rest of their lives. I would remind every medical graduate that you have only one life to live, so enjoy it to the fullest. Try rural medicine, even for a short time and if you are the type of person to fit into that particular lifestyle you will not make as much money as your urban colleagues, but you will be rich and rewarded in many other ways. And, if you decide country practice is not for you, the experience will still make you a better doctor, either as a specialist or as an urban general practitioner.

About the author

J. Cameron MacDonald was born in Sydney, Cape Breton, in 1925, the son of lawyer Finlay MacDonald KC, MP, and Olive Guthrie MacDonald, BLIFTCL, teacher, broadcaster and Shakespearean scholar. Cameron was named after a Roman Catholic Bishop, who has since turned over in his crypt many times.

Despite having educated parents and a happy home, Cameron was a high school dropout, worked as a labourer in the local steel plant open hearth and eventually made his way to St. Francis Xavier University and Dalhousie Medical School.

For five years, he was the only medical doctor on the Digby Islands, 40 miles and a ferry ride from the nearest hospital. He looked after 1,200 people, delivered 57 babies at home with chloroform anaesthesia, along with everything else, and loved the life.

He later specialized in radiology and currently lives with his wife of 58 years in Windsor, Ontario. They have four children and eight grandchildren.

"I chose law, Cam chose medicine. We were both right".
- Neil McKelvey, Past President, Canadian Bar Association

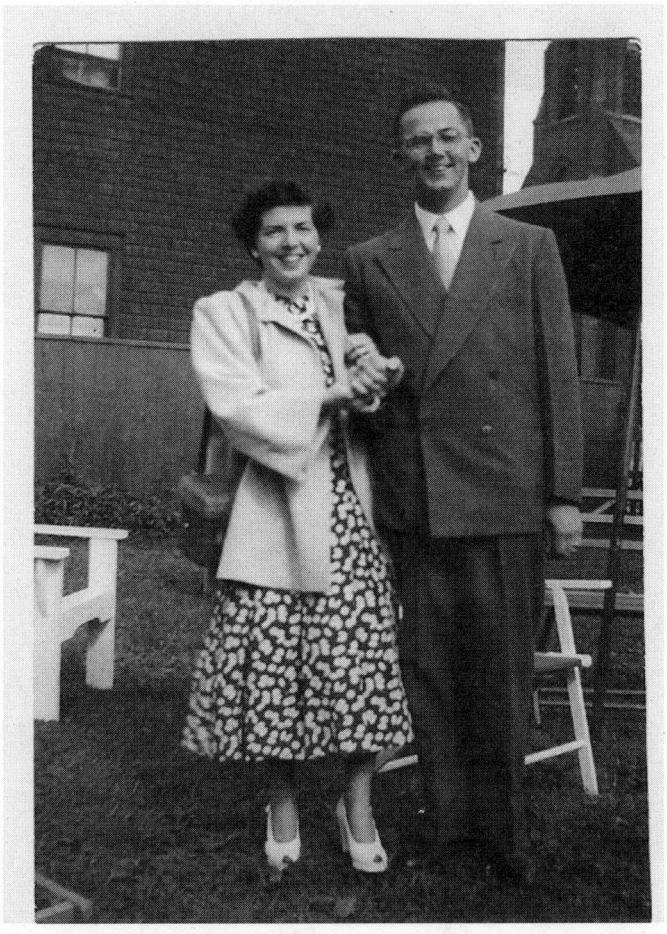

Married, 3rd yr. Medical School

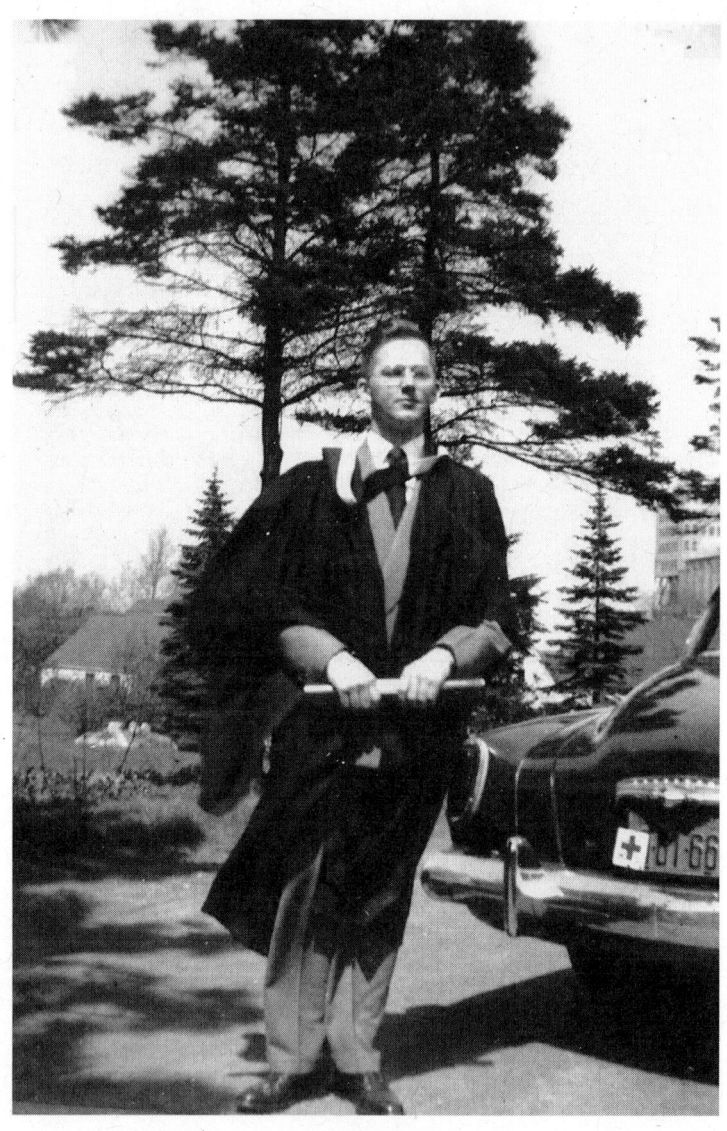

J. Cameron MacDonald, M.D., C.M.
Medical School, Dalhousie University Graduation Day,
May 15, 1951

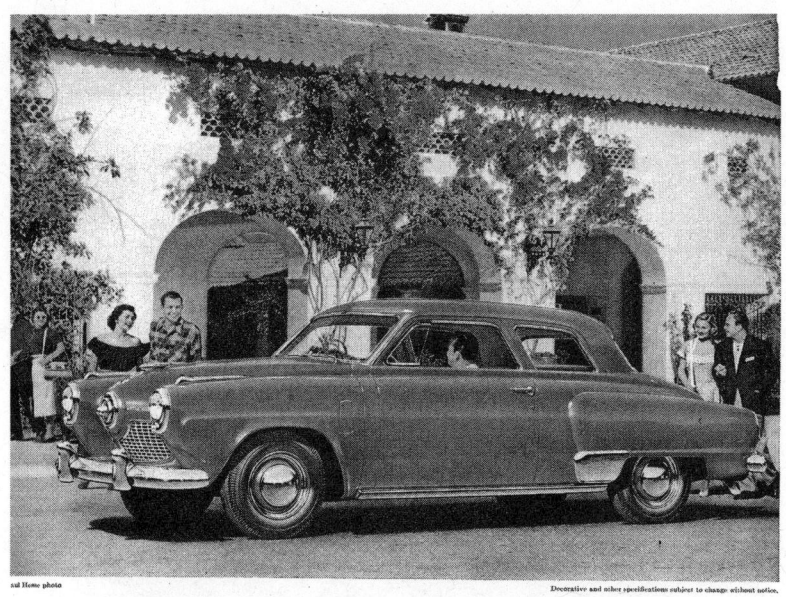

sid Home photo — Decorative and other specifications subject to change without notice.

New driving thrill! 120-horsepower wonder car!

Spectacular Studebaker Commander V-8

A jet-streamed powerhouse on wheels!
New-type high efficiency valve-in-head V-8 engine!
Sensational acceleration! Exceptional thrift!*
A stand-out in quality! A bargain buy!

*Best 8 in actual gas mileage in 1951 Mobilgas Run.
Overdrive, optional at extra cost, was used.

SEE THE THRIFTY STUDEBAKER CHAMPION, TOO...TOP VALUE OF THE TOP 4 LOWEST PRICE CARS

©1951, The Studebaker Corporation, South Bend 27, Indiana, U.S.A.

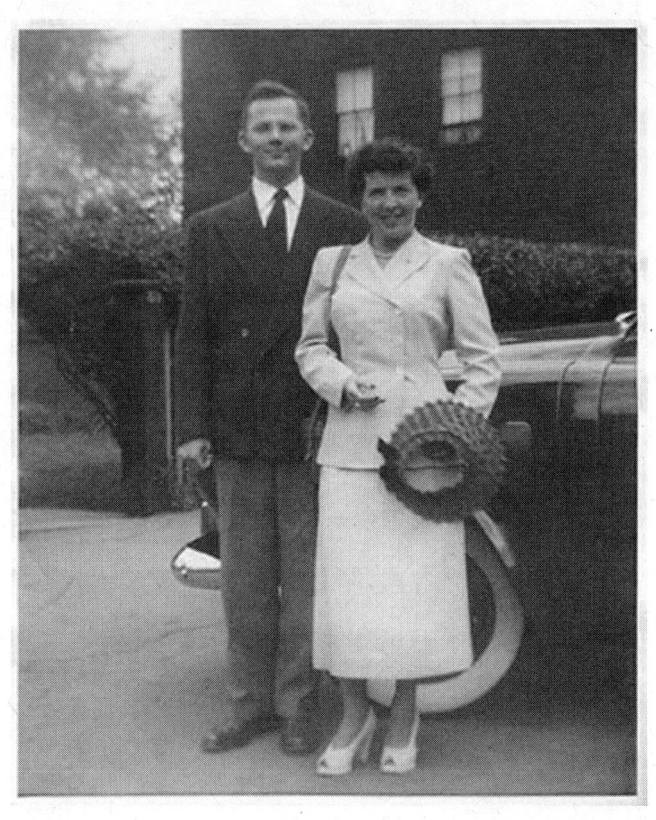

first new car

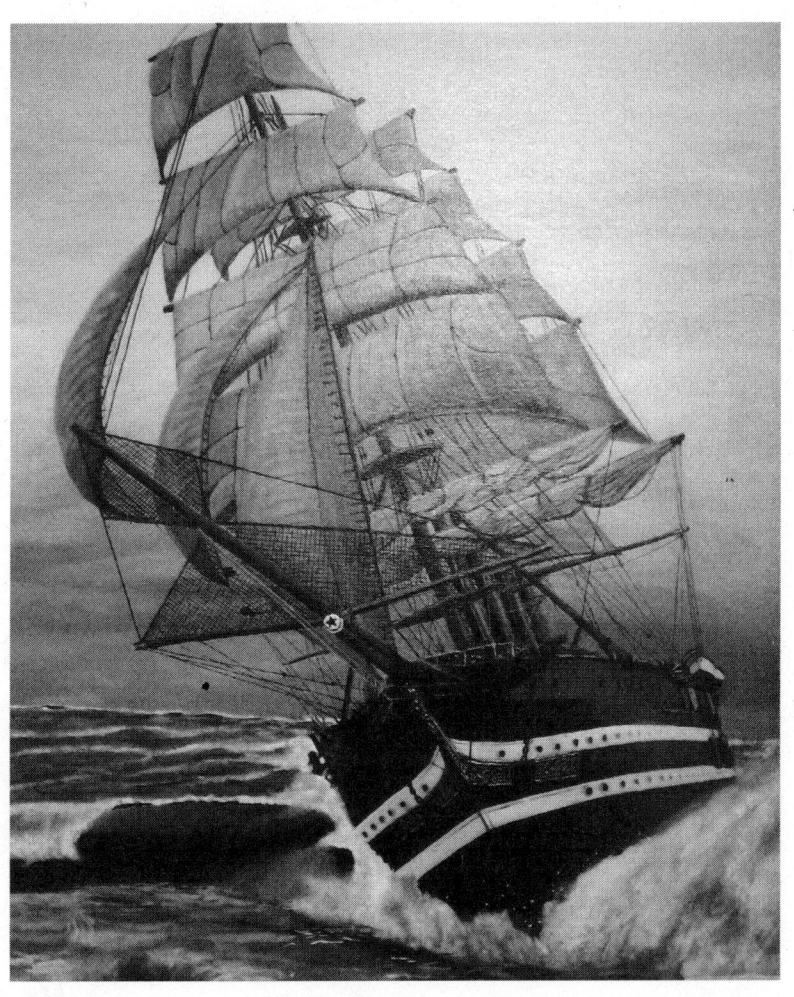

Shipwreck by Rodney Stark

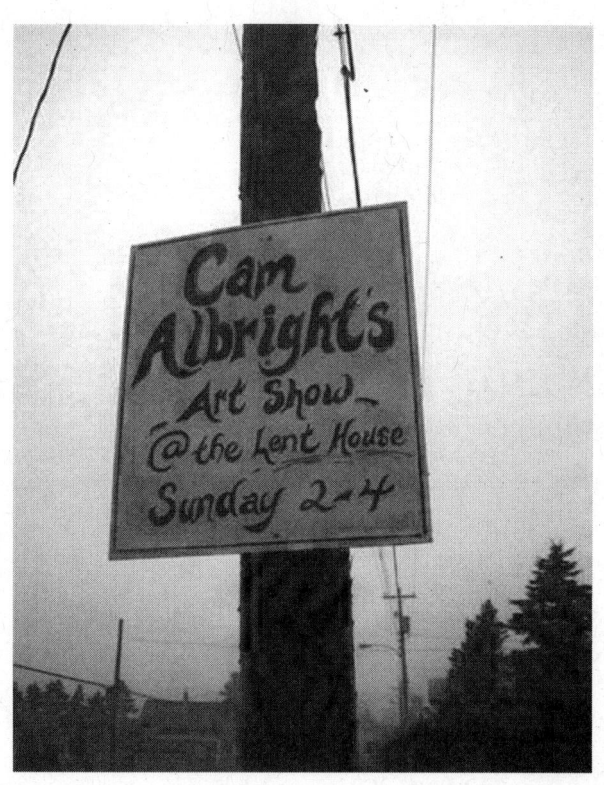

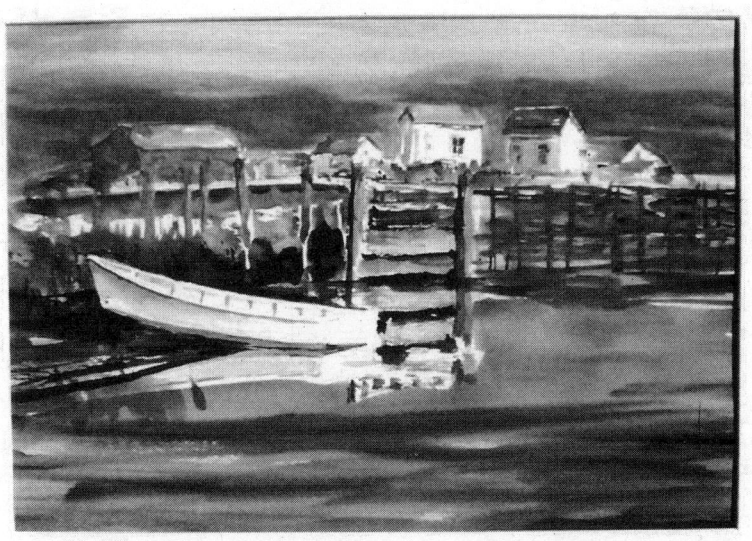

Fish Point Wharf by Cam Albright

Saint John, N.B. Harbour Pilot Boats
on which
Captain William P. Traynor served
1930-1957

David Lynch   1921-1930
(PICTURE NOT AVAILABLE)

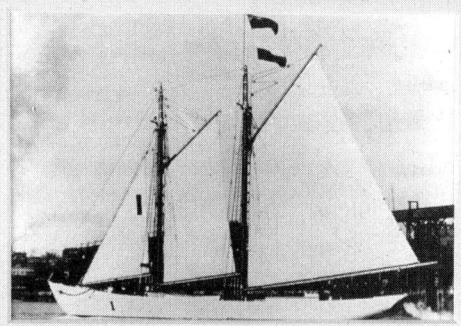

Glooscap   1930-1933

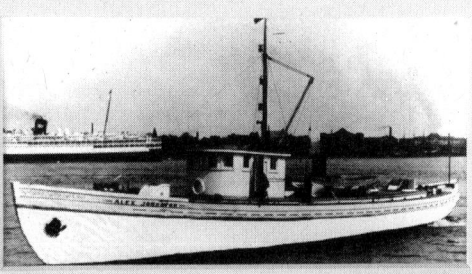

Alex Johnston   1934-1942

Phone 22

FREEPORT, N. S. *April 28* 19 *53*

Freeport

IN ACCOUNT WITH

J. CAMERON MacDONALD, M. D., C. M.

TO PROFESSIONAL SERVICES
AND MEDICINE

may 26 . Delivery Twins | 35 | 00